HEALERS AND ALTERNATIVE MEDICINE

For Chris, Mike and Hazel

Healers and Alternative Medicine

A Sociological Examination

GARY EASTHOPE
University of Tasmania

Gower

Published by
Gower Publishing Company Limited, Gower House,
Croft Road, Aldershot, Hants GU11 3HR, England

and

Gower Publishing Company, Old Post Road,
Brookfield, Vermont 05036, U.S.A.

British Library Cataloguing in Publication Data

Easthope, Gary
  Healers and alternative medicine : a sociological
  examination.
  1. Therapeutic systems——Social aspects
  2. Social medicine
  I. Title
  306'.46   RA418

ISBN 0 566 05098 6

Printed in Great Britain by Blackmore Press, Shaftesbury, Dorset.

Contents

Acknowledgements

This is the most difficult part of the book to write. My debts are enormous and I can never fully repay them.

First and foremost, I must thank all those who allowed me to talk to them and observe them in action. Not only did they give me time but were also kind enough to comment on my descriptions of their healing practices and correct my misunderstandings. It must be realised, however, that the descriptions given in this book remain my own, misunderstandings and all, and that although I have attempted to present the healer's viewpoint, that viewpoint has been edited by me. I would strongly recommend anyone interested in non-medical healing to go and see for themselves. If my experience is a guide they will have a friendly welcome and an interesting time.

Secondly, there are the many colleagues and students who have put up with me talking about 'my healers' during the past years, even encouraging me by providing books, booklists and contacts I otherwise would have been unaware of. I am especially grateful to Peter New who gave me much of his time and ideas, as well as giving me the opportunity to meet some of the many American academics with whom I had corresponded and who shared my interest in marginal medicine. In England I owe much to the members of the seminar that met at our house once a fortnight, probably more than they realise!

Thirdly, there are the many non-academics who, because of their interest in healing, have often made helpful comments on my work and their own experience of doctors and healers. Ciony Miranda in the Philippines is an obvious example of such a person, but there have been many more.

Fourthly, there are the institutions that have supported me. My former university, the University of East Anglia at Norwich, provided helpful small grants (particularly for the trip to Lourdes) and a term's leave of absence, enabling me to travel to Canada. There, McGill University Faculty of Education provided me with a room and secretarial assistance asking little in return, while Concordia University Faculty of Education (where my wife worked) were also extremely helpful.

Several typists have struggled with my writing and I can only express my amazement at their abilities in producing order out of chaos. Four in particular need special praise for work 'beyond the call of duty'; Aileen Pink, Anne Martin, Angie Brooks and Nikki Pullen.

Finally there is my wife Chris and son Michael. My wife has not only supported me by listening (again and again) to my arguments as I tried them out on her and provided me with coffee (another cup has just been drunk as I type this). She also, when I wanted to travel abroad, obtained posts in Canada and the Philippines, enabling me to observe healers while she worked assiduously to support me. Mike helped by being himself, especially when he allowed us to cure his warts by reciting over them, every evening, 'Spot, spot, go away.' The warts went; for him healing worked.

Grateful acknowledgement is also made for permission to reprint extracts from the following:

Between Man and Man by M. Buber, 1947. Reprinted by permission of Routledge and Kegan Paul Ltd; The Church is Healing by M. Wilson, 1966. Reprinted by permission of SCM Publications; Health and Healing in Rural Greece by R. Blum and A. Blum, 1965. Reprinted by permission of Stanford University Press; An Introduction to Medical Sociology edited by D. Tucket, 1976. Reprinted by permission of Chapman and Hall; Knowledge of Illness in a Sepik Society by A.J. Lewis, 1975. Reprinted by permission of Athlone Press Ltd and the London School of Economics; Magic, Science and Religion by S. Malinowski, Macmillan 1948. Reprinted by permission of the Society for Promoting Christian Knowledge; Miracles and Pilgrims by R.C. Finucane, 1977. Reprinted by permission of Dent (J.M.) and Sons Ltd; Mysticism by F.C. Happold, 1963. Reprinted by permission of Faber and Faber; Persuasion and Healing by J.D. Frank, 1963. Reprinted by permission of Johns Hopkins University Press; Physical Control of the Mind by R. Delgado, 1969. Reprinted by permission of Harper & Row Publishers Inc; The Placebo Effect in Healing by M. Jospe. Reprinted by permission of D.C. Heath & Co; 'Psychiatry and Religion' by J. Mathers, 1970. Reprinted by permission of SCM Publications; Purity and Danger by M. Douglas, 1966. Reprinted by permission of Routledge and Kegan Paul Ltd; The Second Genesis by A. Rosenfeld, 1975. Reprinted by permission of Random House; Self and Others by R.D. Laing, 1969. Reprinted by permission of Tavistock Publications Ltd; Watcher on the Hills by R. Johnson. Reprinted by permission of Hodder and Stoughton Ltd; The Root of the Matter by M. Isherwood. Reprinted by permission of Victor Gollancz Ltd.

Introduction

This book describes the work of a selection of healers ranging from the psychic surgeons of the Philippines to those who practise in what was my home town of Norwich, England. By healers is meant those who are practising, or are claiming to practise, healing outside the boundaries of conventional medicine. Not all such practitioners lack medical qualifications, I hasten to add so that you do not turn away with the thought that this is yet another book about 'cranks and weirdos'. In fact it is my argument in this book that these alternative practitioners may have some justification for the claim to heal and that the book might equally well have been entitled 'Do Healers Work?' for this is one of the questions which I try to grapple with in the book. The healers that are described in this book claim to produce results that appear magical — they claim health restored to the incurable and to the chronically ill. They also argue that they achieve these results through the use of nonmaterial means: by utilising forces that are not apparent to the senses, they produce results in the material world. This has been the claim of magicians through the centuries.

What this book sets out to demonstrate is that the claim might be justified and should not be summarily dismissed. At the least their theories and practices represent stimulating challenges to simplistic notions of science, technology, religion, magic and identity. Consideration of those challenges has taken me halfway round the world to the Philippines, where this book begins. It has also taken me on an even more peculiar journey through the pathways of philosophy, psychology, sociology and medicine. My account of these journeys is given in the following pages. Wherever possible I have checked my account of my experiences with those I describe and although they did not always like the account all have agreed to allow me to present my own picture. For that I am profoundly grateful to them. At the same time my interpretation of these experiences remains my own and that interpretation is sometimes contentious, as is inevitable when exploring new intellectual areas. I have tried to bring together a large academic literature on healing in a new set of arguments and tried to express these arguments as simply as possible. To maintain this simplicity I have been forced to relegate many of the supports for my arguments and conclusions to footnotes. This is especially true of the final chapter. I can only ask those who want to find out where I dug out some of my ideas to quarry the footnotes.

The journey I write of started in Norwich and in the fact that I volunteered to teach the Sociology of Religion. I do not like teaching courses unless I research in the same area, for I find research the quickest and surest way to make sense of a new field. So I cast about for a field of research in religion and faith healing sprang to mind, especially as I could find few references to others working in the area. From that beginning I went to a healing centre in Norwich and from there the net spread wider and wider. However, the net was never cast with any particular fish in mind. I just threw it out and was grateful for whatever I pulled in. After studying various groups in Norwich I decided that I needed to go further afield to see if Norwich was at all unusual; and my university generously funded me to travel in England to healing organisations and individuals whose activities I knew only by hearsay. During a sabbatical my wife obtained a visiting post at a Canadian university and then while there took up a consultancy in the Philippines. My net spread world wide.

What fell into it was not only an arbitrary collection of healers and healing organisations but also varied and various data. There was no questionnaire and no research team, merely myself asking people what they were doing, what they thought was happening and observing what was happening myself. The data that resulted from this process were therefore a collection of odd bits and pieces consisting of documents, pamphlets and books given (or sold) to me by the healers, their explanations of themselves - both in these written records and in a taped interview with me - and my observations of where they worked and what they did. For some the data collected in this way was abundant, for others it was a barely adequate minimum.

For a long time I tried to patch this jumble into a whole cloth. The problem was it kept falling apart at the seams. The data was inadequate and anyway the structuring got in the way of an appreciation of the patches of data which were fascinating in themselves. Therefore I present the reader with the bits and pieces so that he can draw his own conclusions. My attempts to stitch parts together are also included. To do more requires a research team of physiologists, doctors, psychologists and sociologists. Perhaps such a team may be formed one day and may manage to make sense of it all - for the present, however, I report the evidence and the partial sense I made of it.

1 The Philippines

The girl screeched with pain as a teenage boy ground a stone again and again into the skin between the fingers of her left hand. Her cries became louder as a man knelt on the linoleum floor by her chair, grasped her bare right foot firmly and pressed a medallion into the skin. When a woman dressed in a white coat attacked her left foot in a similar fashion her screeching turned to sobs. Around these four people the paraffin lamps shone on a roomful of people chattering to each other and preparing food for supper. To the girl the contrast must have been dreamlike. She was being tormented in the middle of a happy party and nobody seemed to notice! She sobbed and pleaded in gasping breaths for them to stop. At last the man did stop but the respite was short, for the others redoubled their efforts, the woman in the white coat transferring her attentions from the left to the right foot.

This small drama is not a description of an interrogation session in a rather brutal spy movie. Nor, as the woman dressed all in white might suggest, is it an operation carried out without anaesthesia. It shows, however, elements of both of these. It was an attempt to deal with a case of bewitchment, a case of witchcraft, in Manila, the major city of the Philippines. It was, for me, a good example of the Filipino concern with witchcraft and one of the most dramatic attempts to deal with it I observed.

Filipinos are ardent believers in witchcraft. This belief is not confined to the uneducated but pervades all sections of their society. A survey amongst students in higher education[1], for example, found that over a quarter claimed to have dreamt of the 'Aswang' (witch) and nearly three quarters feared the howling of dogs which is seen as a warning of 'onitos' (spirits). For most Filipinos their witchcraft beliefs are part of everyday life. Their witches are not funny old women in black hats riding on broomsticks but their neighbours, schoolfriends and colleagues. Life in Manila is harsh and competitive in a manner that is almost impossible for a westerner to imagine. On the streets small boys, no older than seven or eight, dash out in bare feet to sell single cigarettes, newspapers, dusters and towels with

which the drivers of the 'jeepneys', the ubiquitous
decorated steel 'bus' of Manila, mop their sweating faces.
Children scrabble in the earth pushed up by a moving
bulldozer, looking for scraps of metal to sell to supplement
their family's income, risking their lives for a few
coppers. Many never make it into adult life; one in every
thousand Filipino children suffers from third degree
malnutrition which means he is 25 per cent of the body
weight appropriate to his age. Eight year olds look like two
year olds and two year olds look like concentration camp
victims. Those children hustling in the streets may be seven
or eight but they look like five year olds. They are not
starving but they are not adequately fed. Those who succeed
in this desperate scramble for sustenance have to employ
private armies, armed guards to watch over the entrance to
their homes. Armed guards are, in fact, a ubiquitous feature
of Manila and can even be found guarding cheap restaurants.
Coupled with this Dickensian competitiveness of the streets
goes an equally Dickensian reliance on relatives, friends
and neighbours. When you may be starving tomorrow it is good
to have people around you who will share their last crust
with you, just as you would share your last crust with them.
This contrast of the world of the streets, where every man
hustles for himself and tramples his friend underfoot if
necessary, and the world of mutual aid where each man is
expected to help his friend and neighbour, produces a
situation ripe for witchcraft accusations. A successful man
knows his friends are jealous of him and envy him his
success in which they have no share. Thus when he gets ill
or his efforts in business or education fail he puts it down
to their envy and jealousy - their witchcraft which is
dragging him back down. It is therefore not surprising that
over a quarter of those in higher education had dreams of
witchcraft because education, modelled on the American
system, is highly competitive, and, because of the
competitive examination system, it is objectively true that
one man's success is another man's failure. A successful
student is one who has left his family to fend for
themselves while he comes to Manila to study and who has
succeeded over the broken dreams of his former fellow
students whom he has beaten in competitive examination.

What can you do if you are a Filipino and you are ill or
your ventures are not succeeding as well as they should and
you suspect the envy of your intimates is the cause? What
you do is to go and see a healer who can alleviate your
distress. There are many such in Manila. Most parish
churches have a healer who appears one day a week to cope
with the afflictions presented to her. These healers are
usually older women who originally came into Manila from the
country. Often illiterate, they form part of a peasant
tradition in which it was the responsibility of the older
women to pray for the dead, reciting the litany by memory.
One I observed stood at the back of a church after Mass
looking, from her glazed eyes, as though she were in a
trance. As each person approached her she laid hands on
their head, their forehead, their shoulders, their arms and

4

their abdomen in a continuous flowing movement. Each person touched, bowed and kissed her hand before moving away, a continuous stream of over a hundred people. Each encounter took place in silence except for an occasional soft voiced comment from the healer or the supplicant with some individuals directing her hands to a particular part of their body. When the queue of people finally spluttered to an end, the healer just turned and walked into the little vestibule behind her, presumably to reappear the following week.

Obviously such healers play an important role in the life of the parish but they represent only the front line of a more complex phenomena. Some healers, because they are particularly effective at relieving distress or curing bewitchment, acquire a reputation outside their own parish. Some may even gain international reputations because what they do is spectacular and fits in better with western ideas of healing. I was able to observe two such healers during my stay in Manila. The first, from which the short account with which this chapter began was taken, was a woman working within the Catholic tradition, the religious faith of most Filipinos. The second, a man, was a psychic surgeon operating in a spiritualist tradition.

ST NINO

Mrs Fabiana Macaraan is the mother in law of Ciony's first cousin. Ciony was my wife's chaperone and she had agreed to introduce me to Mrs Macaraan. Ciony had been trained as a healer by Mrs Macaraan and she explained being a healer to me in these terms:

> You can't heal unless you are purified in thought. I can only heal when the spirit descends on me. It's dangerous if you are not purified. There would be an intermingling of your thoughts and spirit thoughts - it can lead to confusion. If you are not purified then evil spirits can capture you. If you are purified then the good spirit can capture your mind. It's a race between the good and the bad spirit to capture you. The instrument should be a pious person but need not be Catholic. If you have a spirit in you, as long as you are treating you do not feel fatigue, thirst or hunger.

We went to Pagasa Road in Quezon City, a section of metropolitan Manila, to see this healer. Ciony saw the name of the road as very significant. It means 'hope' in Tagalog, the principal language of the Philippines. This concern with the significance of names was not confined to Ciony; people were fascinated by our name 'Easthope' which becomes 'Pagasang Silangon' in Tagalog and read into it great significance, especially as my wife had come to teach teachers of handicapped children. In the uncertain world in which Filipinos live, signs which suggest better things are eagerly sought just as they were in Tudor England (Thomas, 1973).

Mrs Macaraan was never referred to by that name but by the term 'Nanang Fabing' (Mother Dear) or as 'Mahal na St Nino' (our dear infant Jesus), when she was possessed by the infant Jesus. To reach her house we took a long hot journey by bus and then a jeepney which dropped us off at the corner of the street. The street was beaten earth with sugar cane growing at the corner, where bare footed children played. The housing was closely packed but it was not a shanty settlement. By the time we arrived it was dark and the narrow passageway which led into Nanang Fabing's room was lit by an oil lamp. In the passageway people were lined up, sitting or standing on both sides. I was taken straight past these patiently waiting people, with Ciony giving a nod of the head to a man sitting on a seat by the door, and immediately introduced to the healer who blessed Ciony and gave her a communion wafer and then blessed me and also gave me a communion wafer.

The room in which Nanang Fabing sat was about nine feet by six feet with painted wooden walls. The light was dim but adequate and came from paraffin lamps. In this tiny room there were more than twenty people. The right hand side of the room consisted of a curtain behind which a few women were busy preparing food and placing it on a table. Also behind the curtain, at the end of the room, there was a steep narrow flight of stairs. For most of my observation of the healer I squatted on this staircase looking through a large gap in the curtain and dripping sweat as I scribbled.

As I entered the room the focus of attention was on the healer. Nanang Fabing was a small woman, even by Filipino standards (where even the men are, on average, only about five feet four inches in height), sitting on a large swivel chair and dressed in red trousers and a white blouse. No one else was allowed to sit in the chair at any time. If you were foolish enough to do so, I was told, you would get a pain in your body. Around her neck was a microphone attached to a battery operated tape recorder which occupied a small table, above which was a collection box. Next to this table, sitting against the passageway, was a boy who supervised the tape recorder. His job was to record the words she spoke when she became St Nino, the infant Jesus. Next to him sat a young woman in her thirties, dressed all in white. She, I was told, came from the same rural area as the major healer and like her was also illiterate, but in her case she became possessed by the Virgin Mary. The small area of the concrete floor on which these three were located was covered with linoleum, and before stepping on the linoleum people removed their shoes. (I blundered on it in my sandals, not realizing my mistake until later.)

Behind Nanang the wall was decorated with religious pictures: a crucifix and a Madonna and Child lit from inside were to her right; above that was a lit Jesus as a crowned

child; above her head there was a lit Virgin Mary, while to
her left there was a lit Christ. There were numerous other
sacred pictures and objects on the walls of the room. Some
of these were said to have special significance. One of the
pictures of Christ is known as the 'eye' portrait and it is
believed that if you meditate by focusing upon it you see
visions. This picture can also obviate the need to confess
to a priest. If you are sincere in your confession to it, I
was told, you can feel the crucifix in it perspiring and you
are forgiven.

One object in particular just stated simply '5 October
1973'. This celebrates the day Nanang was given her power.
She received her power after being given visions of the
infant Jesus. Initially she resisted these visions because
she wanted to look after her son, who was the last of her
eight children at home, by continuing to work as a laundry
woman for which she earned 400 pesos a month (approximately
25 pounds but a good sum by Filipino standards; teachers are
paid about 600 pesos a month). She became paralyzed, but
when the next apparition appeared and she agreed to become a
healer, the paralysis left her. When the spirit descends on
her she speaks like a child. Sometimes this is a four year
old child and sometimes a twelve year old. She also
occasionally is possessed by other spirits such as Jahweh
and Mary.

She treats people every day, except Wednesday. On the
first Friday of each month her disciples come and have their
power renewed. The disciples formed the majority of those in
the room when I entered. The women were in red dresses and
the men were in red trousers and a white T shirt with a thin
red collar. They are all devotees of the Black Nazarene and
this is the uniform of such devotees. The Black Nazarene is
a dark wooden statue of Jesus on the cross. It is normally
kept in Quiapo church, in the poorest area of central
Manila, but is brought out once a year in procession. During
the procession thousands of young men struggle to touch the
statue for to touch it brings luck for the year. Usually
some die in this fervent struggle. Devotees of different
shrines wear different uniforms, e.g. the devotees of the
Shrine of Our Lady of Lourdes (which is a Filipino 'copy' of
the famous Lourdes Shrine, see Chapter 3) wear a white
uniform with a blue sash and a small lace cap. Filipinos in
general seem to like to wear uniform whenever they can, and
even teachers and teacher trainers also have uniforms.
Nanang's treatment is free and you can donate whatever you
like. Many people donate food and that is what the women
behind the curtain were preparing for later distribution to
everyone there. Others donated the religious objects hung
about the room.

The proceedings continued after my entry with her
disciples going up to her one by one. To each of them, as
she had done for Ciony and myself, she held her hands up in
blessing, gave each a wafer on their tongue then blessed the
individual, held their hands in her palms and closed their

hands by clasping them. After she had blessed them all she began to rock back and forth and mutter. Ciony assured me she was now speaking as St Nino. I could detect no change in the tone of her voice although apparently her grammatical construction was of a four year old child in her own dialect. (There are 49 dialects in the Philippines.) The woman dressed in white knelt before her and was touched on the head, and then had her hands held by St Nino. After this the woman in white began to breathe deeply and clasped her hands in the prayer position so often depicted in religious statues and pictures of the Virgin Mary. She suddenly pushed her hands out, crossing and recrossing them (to drive away the evil spirits, I was informed). Then she blessed everyone with hands that were trembling, and said, 'I am happy for everyone here, typhoons will be coming this year, and I have given you candles to light.' She then sat back in an obvious trance, her head thrown back and her arms along the chair arms. At this point St Nino said in Tagalog (the dominant dialect of the region and the Philippines) and in English (for my benefit) 'Hello everybody. All right. Eating time now. Chow time.'

While everyone was eating, except the healers, and people were moving in and out of the serving area both St Nino and the Blessed Virgin Mary began to treat people. This treatment was somewhat difficult to observe as both St Nino and the Blessed Virgin Mary were treating at the same time. In addition the boy by the tape recorder sometimes treated people as did some of the disciples. None the less most of the treatment was undertaken by St Nino and the Blessed Virgin Mary. The Blessed Virgin Mary mainly used a gesture of throwing something away from people while St Nino used a variety of methods. Nor did all the people come to be healed. They came for a variety of reasons: to get their money blessed, or their purse blessed so they would never be poor, to get their pens blessed before an examination, to have stones, medals and beads blessed so that they could treat other people, to ask for intelligence for a backward child, to get predictions about their future, or to get advice about problems, to find out the sex of their unborn child, to have themselves blessed against witchcraft, to be freed from a witchcraft curse, to be cured of sterility, to get the drugs prescribed by a doctor blessed, to find a lost object by giving the name of the person they thought had stolen it [2]. Some people queued up several times to see different healers for different problems. The healers' methods of blessing and healing varied a good deal. They healed by holding the person's head and throwing away the sickness, by holding the eyes of the afflicted and breathing upon them, by massaging and then throwing away, by dropping pure water - after blessing it - on to the eyes or the throat from a cotton wool pad, by treating with alcohol a sore tongue or the cut on the foot of a child, by making people drink the blessed water while the healer pressed the side of their throat as they did so to cure them of phlegm (there's a very high T.B. rate in Manila), by stroking and throwing away, by chopping with the side of the hand or two fingers at the arm or head of the patient and by kneading the abdomen. These various healing practices were done extremely rapidly and it was not always possible to find out which particular method was used for which affliction. Nonetheless my impression was that about a third had come for some form of blessing, another third for eye afflictions or throat afflictions (a not surprising occurrence given the polluted air of Manila and the crowded living conditions) and the rest from a variety of causes. One case was particularly interesting - a case of witchcraft.

A young girl in her early twenties dressed in slacks, sloppy shirt and thong sandals asked for help from one of the healers (the young boy operating the tape recorder). She was an attractive girl, large by Filipino standards. She thought she was bewitched. She was married and had three children and kept on getting pains. These she attributed to her husband's former common law wife who was jealous of her because she was very industrious. She had been treated twice before. My informants told me, none the less, that a successful cure of witchcraft was rare these days and that I was lucky to be observing one. One of the healers looked at her little fingers and diagnosed that she was bewitched because one finger was longer than the other. Two men then began to treat the girl. One of the men was the boy who operated the tape recorder and the other was a disciple. The boy pressed a holy stone hard between the fingers of her left hand while the man pressed a religious medallion between her toes. While they did this they told her she was bewitched. The girl was in agony from this treatment and screeched. They asked her to bear the pain because they wanted to catch the spirits in her body. A woman healer, the Blessed Virgin Mary, joined them and pushed an object into the girl's left foot. The girl was now sobbing and beseeching them to stop. Ciony told me that that was the evil spirit speaking and asking them not to punish it any more because it would not do it again. While all this drama was taking place other people nearby behind the curtains were ignoring it, happily cutting up food for supper for the healers later and chatting away to each other. St Nino then intervened and grabbed the girl's right hand saying 'Enough, enough. Why are you bewitching this girl?' The girl gave no response but as the objects were removed she stopped yelling and slumped in her chair. They asked her to wake up from her trance and first the boy and then St Nino slapped her on the forehead. When she emerged from the trance state she was given a drink of water and the tension in the room eased. St Nino told the others that they must be careful when doing this treatment and check for the pulse and heartbeat because if overdone it can kill the person. The girl looked very relaxed and everyone was kind to her and smiled at her for the rest of the evening.

After this event the boy told me his story (in English):

When I was still studying medical technology I topped the exams. Someone was jealous. I was bewitched.

9

My lips were bleeding without any scientific cause.
Medicine was no help. I came here to be treated and I
was healed. When you are treating for bewitchment it
is not always the case that you talk to the spirit.
When you are strong he (the spirit) can't get into
the body and when you are in pain he will remove (the
affliction) he gave to the person. Now, the black
Nazarene descends on me. Sometimes when I'm praying I
feel I'm floating in the air, I feel weightless.

The session was closed with the various healers and
disciples treating each other, the girl possessed by the
Blessed Virgin Mary sleeping in a chair. When I left, supper
was being served to the healers, who had not eaten earlier
with everyone else.

A PSYCHIC HEALER

This healer, Alex Orbito, was also found by Ciony but with
much more difficulty. She found him, in fact, just before I
left the country and took me to his house. To get there we
took a bus. Unfortunately it was rush hour and the bus was
so crowded that the man standing next to my seat could not
even stand upright but had to lean over at an angle which
forced me to bend my head sideways. The result was an
extremely stiff neck. By the time we arrived I felt in need
of a healer. He was not there, however, as he was on a
working visit to Singapore. We took the telephone number and
on his return I was able to visit him by myself.

The detached house had large iron gates at the entrance.
It was situated in a road behind a large Iglesia Christi
church. (These churches are found all over Luzon, the main
island of the Philippines, and are all built to the same
pattern - Disneyland castle style converted to Gothic church
in white concrete - whatever their size). Inside the gates,
which had a small door set in them, was a tiny walled
courtyard occupied by a car which took up about a third of
the space, and garden tables and chairs in wrought iron. To
the left of the entrance across the courtyard there was an
extension to the house. This was the room where the healing
took place and people were standing around waiting for the
French windows to it to be opened.

When they did I followed the others into the room which
was about 40 feet long by 20 feet wide. Along the left hand
wall were built-in bookcases with only a few books on them,
and the opposite wall had windows covered in lace curtains.
Most of the white marble floor was covered by wooden chairs
arranged in rows facing toward the far wall. At that end of
the room there was a door into the rest of the house on the
left and to the right a large table, the top of which was
covered in a white plastic tablecloth pinned down around the
edge with drawing pins over a green cloth, which hung down
to hide the legs. On the wall behind the table there were
three objects: a picture of God the Father painted on wood,

10

one of the Virgin Mary in 'stained glass' and a larger
central banner in silk. The banner had a picture of Jesus
with a prominent heart in its centre above which were the
words 'Grace of the Holy Spirit' and below was written:

> Carazon de Amor
>   de
> Esperito Santo
> St.James v. 14-15
> Rev.Alex Orbito   (The Healer)
> 93 Sgt Catulos Q.City   (His address)

I was approached by a 'guard' who asked what I was doing
here. He also approached a German who had come for treatment
for his chin. We were at this time the only two 'white'
people there, although more arrived later. The guard
proceeded to explain what was about to happen:

> There will be a bible reading, this is anaesthesia.
> People clean themselves...wash themselves so
> they are spiritually clean, mind, conscience and
> body prepared. This is the work of God. If possible
> you must clean yourself. With the power he knows if
> you are clean, then...when Alex recites the
> prayer from the Bible and from Psalm 51 (the
> prayer of repentance) he receives the Holy Spirit.
> Then he will bless the water and oil on the
> table. After the blessing he is going to heal. He
> tells people who are cured to go to the doctor.
> They are improved, they are healed, and the
> doctor is amazed to know. He lets some take
> blood clots to be examined by the doctor.

While he was telling me this a man was standing at the
front of the room with a Bible in his hand expounding in
dialect to the audience. The guard then took me through the
door to meet Alex. He was an unprepossessing man, of slim
build, looking somewhat red eyed and tired. He told the
guard to take me back and ensure I got a good position so
that I could take photographs. On my return to the main room
the guard asked the German if he also would like to be near
the front and he came and stood next to me to the right of
the table which abutted the right hand wall of the room. I
initially stood by the door behind the table but I was told
that this was not allowed. White people were definitely
given easier access to the healer and were treated first or
given special attention at the end.

By this time there were approximately thirty people of all
ages in the room, the women outnumbering the men. The
atmosphere, with all the people in it, had become hot and
humid which the small fan in the roof did little to
dissipate. People were fanning themselves as they waited for
the next stage of the proceedings, for the man expounding
with a Bible in his hand had stopped.

The next stage began when a young woman, speaking in

English, said, 'Let us start with our prayers. Please stand.' Then she began reading from Psalm 51: 'Wash me thoroughly from my iniquity...in sin did my mother conceive me...wash me and I shall be whiter than snow...hide thy face from my sins.' This was followed by the Lord's Prayer. She then told the congregation to sit and not to worry about numbers. (There was a rack of plastic numbers, each person took one as they entered the room. This is the normal way to cope with queues in North America and presumably had been adopted by Filipinos although I had never seen it used elsewhere in Manila.)

Alex then entered holding a Bible upright between his palms and wearing normal attire: a short sleeved barong tagalog (the embroidered shirt worn by most Filipinos) and trousers. He then began to lecture to the audience using both Tagalog and English (for my benefit?). His style of delivery was rhythmic and he used his hands and arms economically. He told them where he had visited - America, Saudi Arabia, Malaysia - and referred to the Europeans present as evidence of his fame. He stressed 'this is spiritual healing. You must transfer your material mind to the spiritual level...there are two kinds of body, the material body and the spiritual body.' He then went on to talk of his recent visit to Singapore and said, 'The tradition of the Chinese people is of another kind but they are believers in spiritual healing. There are many kinds of tribes of people who believe in spiritual healing.' He then went on to expound the idea that God the Father came from the West, God the Son from the Middle East and now God the Spirit has come from the Far East; 'God the Father and Son are finished. We are now in the time of the Spirit.' He went on: 'I'm not God. I'm only the vessel of the Spirit. The Spirit is in me.' He continued by talking of the two kinds of matter again before saying, 'I give the Filipino three days, American man Monday, Wednesday, Sunday and Friday. The Filipinos are my neighbours, that is why I give only three days.' He concluded his exposition by telling of cures that had occurred with Australians and stressed positive thinking: 'If you know how to smile the world will smile too, to you.'

While he was expounding his helpers were busy. There were three of them, two young girls in their twenties and an older man in his forties. They had been arranging on the table in front of him a pillow, three bottles, two plastic tupperware containers and a carafe of water. In addition, one of the girls dropped cottonwool into saucers full of a clear liquid by the bookshelves and put a small towel next to the pillow along with some cottonwool.

At the end of his exposition Alex bent over the Bible held tightly upright between his palms. His helpers, who had sat down after their preparations, stood up again, although the congregation remained seated. His hands began shaking and he murmured prayers. He then passed his hand over the bottles on the table while a girl helper held an open Bible over his

hands. When this short ritual was concluded the bottles were
taken off the table and the saucers brought over. Alex
announced that those with neck or head problems should sit
on the chair, which was behind the left of the table near
the door, while those with stomach or back problems should
come to the table.

People lined up quickly and Alex began to treat them. A
woman climbed on the table and lay down on her stomach. Her
clothes had already been loosened by one helper and another
stood with a saucer held in her hand. Alex put his hand on
her back where blood suddenly showed and then he removed a
blood clot which he dropped in a saucer. As soon as he had
done this he turned to a woman sitting on the chair and
repeated the process with her neck. While he was treating
her the first woman had her back swabbed clean by a helper
and climbed down from the table, allowing another woman,
this time with a breast problem, to climb up and be waiting
for immediate treatment when Alex turned back to the front.
As he did this the woman on the chair had her neck swabbed
clean by a helper. This rapid pattern of table/chair
table/chair, table/chair continued for some time. As he
probed at people he grimaced and gave a picture of painful
concentration. When he pressed there was a popping sound
shortly before he removed the blood clots. People were
granted as much modesty as was possible in the
circumstances, e.g. a man treated for piles had his backside
covered with a sheet and women were likewise screened in the
genital area.

Suddenly he stopped treating and left the room. One of the
helpers told me that he had a break when he felt tired. The
people waited patiently and quietly for his return and a
helper slopped out a bloody bucket. After about five minutes
he returned to find a child on the table with the parents
waiting with it. One of the helpers asked the parents what
was wrong with the child, who was crying bitterly, and told
Alex. This was a common feature of the treatment in that
Alex didn't talk much but relied on his helpers to find out
the complaint and then tell him. He didn't remove any blood
from the child but just put his hands either side of the
child's head. The helper (who I was later told was a medical
doctor) spent a long time talking to the child's father.
Alex then continued the same table/chair sequence as he had
been doing before his break. At about ten-thirty, when he
had been treating for about one hour, the French windows at
the back of the room were closed and the people left outside
peered through them as the final few were treated. These
included a man with toothache, who had his tooth removed by
Alex working it loose with his hands, and the German who,
unlike the Filipino patients, got instructions from Alex to
close his eyes and pray while he rubbed the chin which had
an infection.

The session finally ended at ten forty-five with Alex
slumped in his chair. He was immediately questioned by an
American about where his power came from. He asked: 'Why is

13

it important to you?   I'm tired.' But he went on to say he
had a spirit guide and his power was the force of that
spirit.   If the force of the sick cells of the body was less
than the force of the spirit then there was dissolution of
the cells. When he removed his hands from the patient there
was cohesion again and no scar was left. The objects he
removed were 'objective materialisations of the negative
forces of sickness and disease.' He went on to point out
that there are fake healers. The questioning went on and he
said that he kept track of patients but had no idea of the
cure rate: 'In Europe and Singapore it is 80 per cent cured
not a 100 per cent. I'm only the guardian of the spirit.' At
the time he treats them he believes all are cured. He is a
believer in witchcraft and said 'concentration of good
influences from the mind heals, concentration of evil brings
disease.' He has to keep healing because 'if I stop healing
I become ill. I do operations everyday.' The house we were
in was rented and he claimed that he'd like to give away all
his money. Such money as he did collect was for a chapel to
be built for his organisation in the provinces which
includes mediums and clairvoyants as well as healers.

    Alex Orbito is probably typical of most psychic surgeons.
By his own account[3] he 'was born in...a far flung province
(as a) child of a tenant farmer...the youngest in a family
of fourteen of which six are still alive. (His) parents are
not only farm workers, they, too, are the healers in (their)
barrio and are considered among the founders of the
spiritualist movement in the Philippines. He belongs to the
'Ilocano Tribe (and) it is this tribe to which the majority
of the known spiritual healers and the founders of the
spiritualist movement in my country belong. I became aware
of the healing power working through me only when I reached
the age of fourteen...that is, when I started to have
recurrent dreams.' He began healing when a neighbour's
mother called him to heal her paralysis after seeing him
heal her in a dream.

        My mother and I accompanied our neighbour's son to
    their home. As soon as his mother saw me...she
    exclaimed...'It's you, yes, it's you I saw in my
    dream' and she started to cry. Without saying a word
    I moved close to her and picked up a bottle of
    coconut oil laying on top of a small table beside the
    bed. And like in my dream I knelt beside her and said
    a short but earnest prayer. I didn't even realise
    that tears were rolling down my cheek as I massaged
    her limbs. Then I took her hands and held them
    between my palms and I told her to stand. Without
    any help she moved her legs down the side of the bed.
    I pulled her up and when she was standing I commanded
    her to walk. And before the startled eyes of her son
    and my mother, she did! Thus, started my healing
    ministry.

    In fact he shortly after left home and took odd jobs
ending up as a photographer only to go to jail accused of

14

stealing the equipment. In jail he prayed and heard a voice which said, 'Fear not my son. I will help you. But promise me that you will go home and continue using the power in your hands...' After the third time he heard the voice he vowed that he would and was released the next day because someone else confessed to the crime. After leaving the jail he did not go home. He was then stricken with fever and a voice came again saying, 'My son, why have thou forsaken me? Repent, follow my command!' He did and the fever left him.

Other healers tell of similar backgrounds: Antonio C. Agpuoa, the most famous, is also from an obscure country barrio, and discovered his gift when he was nine years old, as is Alex Espino, who started as an assistant to Agpuoa. So to is Placido Palitayan who was an assistant to another healer called Gonzales, whose clients he took over when Gonzales died. All of these men, who are now very rich, insist like Espino that 'The knowledge and practice of psychic surgery is not taught. It comes as a gift from above.'

Most, if not all, healers belong either to the Filipino Christian Church or the Union Esperitista Cristiana, and Orbito claims 'that it is not healing alone, or attending to sick people which occupies my time and efforts but work for these organisations.' Thus

the present breed of healers...call themselves 'spirit' or 'missionary healers'. Firstly, they claim that they are merely instruments of spirit entities who perform the actual healing. Secondly, in the case of missionary healers, particularly, it is because they are missionary priests and doing healing is part of their work as clergymen.

As Alex Orbito says:

When I start healing a patient, I am completely attuned with my spirit guide...I virtually become a 'medium' through which the divine healing of God reaches out into the malignant tissue in the patient's body...in that state of attunement, my hands discharge magnetic vibrations that extract the malignant tissues out from the patient's body (but) the primary mission of healing...is not the elimination of physical ailments, but to promote inner awareness, sense of spiritual attachment and personal fellowship with God.

The church to which Orbito belongs, the Union Esperitista, has a complex hierarchy of membership. They believe only in communicating with spirits at the highest realm of the spirit world and do not, as western spiritualists do, communicate with relatives or friends. This communication with spirits is achieved through a 'speaking medium' (Medium parlente) who acts as a channel for the spirits, who speak through him. However, he can only act as a medium in the presence of the elders of the church and a 'vigilant medium' (medium vigente). The vigilant medium has the gift of perceiving whether or not the speaking medium is truly in contact with the spirit world by observing a ray of light coming from the top of the speaking medium's head or by some other appearance of spirit. Progression within the movement is thus from ordinary membership to speaking medium and then to vigilant medium. There is, however, one further step on the ladder and that is into the role of 'operating medium' (medium operador) and these are the psychic surgeons.

There are probably about twenty five psychic surgeons in the Philippines. They are found only on the main island, Luzon, and appear to have begun their practice some forty years ago as part of the Union Esperitista which was itself founded in 1903. They almost certainly began, like witch doctors in Africa, by removing rusty nails or corn husks from the bodies of those they treated, such objects being seen as the material manifestation of the malignancy of witchcraft. The influence of western medicine, and especially western surgeons, may have led to the substitution of organic material for nails and corn husks. A point suggestive of this interpretation is that the centre of psychic surgery is Baguio City, the former administrative capital of the American rulers of the Philippines.

Psychic surgeons are especially popular with visitors from outside the Philippines, many of whom have never thought of witchcraft and would be appalled to discover that those operating upon them are removing not diseased organs but manifestations of personal malignancy, or witchcraft. People pour in because the psychic surgery is so spectacular, fits in so well with western notions of medical practice, and because they are desperate. One Belgian visitor explained:

> I guess you can call our coming here our last hope, our last card...I am willing to try anything just so my wife can be cured...You've got a lot of hopeless cases here, a lot of people clutching at straws and hoping that their session with Filipino faith healers will be fruitful. You know, when a man is very sick and he has been given only a few months to live, he'll try anything, see anyone, go any place in the hope of being healed.

Well are they healed? Discussion of this point will come up again and again in this book. Such discussion comes back to two debates, time after time, whether we are talking of Filipino healers, the phenomena of Lourdes, or the introduction of a new drug to cure cancer. These two debates can be expressed as: What do we mean by healed; what is success? and Are the methods used effective?

These may seem similar questions. However, they do place the emphasis on different aspects of healing. The first question places emphasis on the outcome of the healing. The second places emphasis upon the technique itself and this distinction can be useful in helping us sort out what is a complex phenomena.

Let us take the last question first - are the methods effective? Are these healers actually cutting people open with their bare hands and removing diseased organs? The answer, disappointingly for many who go in hope, ·is that they are not. They are practising a very skilled act which closely resembles the sleight-of-hand of a stage magician. A Jesuit priest told me of one healer who apparently burst boils on the arm without touching the patient. He had taken doctors to see the phenomena and they could not explain it. It was only when he took a stage magician that the event was explained. The healer had mica concealed under his nails and when he first handled the arms of the patient he scored the boil with this mica without bursting it. Then, later, the healer held one hand in the air away from the boil while squeezing the patient's hand with his other hand. The patient responded to this squeeze by squeezing back which made the muscles on his arm move and the boil burst. Film evidence, utilising slow motion techniques, has demonstrated similar tricks with other healers. The blood and organic matter removed has also been analysed and demonstrated to be of animal, not human origin. One healer's assistant even reported in a Filipino newspaper how her employer would buy such things at the early morning market.

In spite of such evidence many still believe in these healers, putting down the evidence of faked operations as momentary lapses on the part of the healer; even asserting that such lapses only emphasize the extraordinary nature of the 'real' phenomena:

> Healers' condition is not constant: on certain days some healers can produce nothing - especially if they have indulged in sexual excesses. Some healers go through long periods when they cannot work at all as a consequence of loose living, money worries, family problems and the like. Then they may resort to faked operations with dried animal blood or dyes, as the skilled observer can tell at a glance. When they regain control, their powers return in full. The fact that some healers now and then engage in simple sleight-of-hand while at other times performing extraordinary material-isations is clear proof to me of the authenticity of the phenomena.

People continue to believe because those treated do often appear to get better. As a Baguio doctor said,

> I'd say that for every one patient who gets cured or believes he has been cured, there are six who leave Baguio with the same ailments they had when they first came here. But then I have yet to run across a patient who, after a healing session with the faith healers, says outright that he has not been cured or

17

he has been the victim of a hoax. Maybe this could be explained in this way: since these people spent so much money just to come and rested all their hopes on being cured, it is very hard to expect them to say that their trip has been a totally fruitless one.

He went on to say that he what he hears is 'we've improved' or 'we're getting better'. When he was asked if there was any basis for these assertions he replied, 'In many cases perhaps none medically but who am I to tell a sick person that it's not true that he has been cured, he has improved or that he is on his way to recovery.'

The doctor's comment returns us to the first question I asked. What do we mean by healed; what do we mean by success? If patients go away convinced they are better, are they not healed? Anyway, the psychic surgeons are not primarily concerned with physical healing, their 'primary mission of healing...is not the elimination of physical ailments but to promote inner awareness, sense of spiritual attachment and personal fellowship with God'. They are not especially concerned with physical ailments but with spiritual health. There are different notions of health in operation here and different ideas of what it means when we say someone is ill. For most orthodox medicine the criteria for judging illness is a change in a person's body and health is a normal body regardless of how the individual concerned thinks about himself. If he continues to claim illness when the doctor can find nothing wrong with him, he is classed as a hypochondriac and thus dismissed from serious consideration. For most unorthodox healers, on the other hand, the criteria for judging illness is a change in a person's spirit or mind and health is an attitude of mind not a state of the body. The most extreme exponents of this unorthodox view are Christian Scientists who deny the reality of the material world. It is, however, a view shared by many healers and leads to a situation where death can be seen as a triumph of health!. 'The world regards death as the ultimate failure and defeat. Death is the ultimate healing. The ministry of healing opens the way to a marvellous and radiant death' as the chaplain at one healing centre expressed it.

To set out the two extremes in this manner may make for easier understanding, but fuller comprehension requires a more complex picture. To draw up that picture we have to look at ideas about the cause of illness. These ideas can be put into three categories:

1. Illness is a result of an invasion of the person by disruptive forces. These forces can be seen as being wilful, for example, they can be seen as spirits or witches, or they can be seen as entirely without will, for example germs and viruses.

2. Illness is a result of disharmony inside the individual. This disharmony can be seen as a spiritual

18

or mental disharmony such as implied in the Chinese
idea of superfluity of yin or yang. Or it can be a
physical disharmony usually expressed by the mechanical
notion of disequilibrium and a disturbance of
homeostasis.
3.   Illness is a result of a disturbance in the environment
     of the individual, a disturbance which seriously
     affects his functioning in a normal manner. This
     disturbance can be material disruption of the
     environment such as that created by industrial waste or
     it can be social such as a broken marriage.

These different notions of illness imply different ideas
of healing and health. If illness is an invasion then
healing must consist of repelling the invader and healing
practices are those that try to attack the invader and expel
it. For bewitchment the healer torments the individual so
that the invading spirit or witch abandons the person
because life becomes too uncomfortable for it. The healer
exorcizes the demon. For viral or bacterial invasions the
healer gives noxious medicines to purge the invaders out of
the body. In both the emphasis is upon an attack on the
invader and the individual who has been involved is
relatively unimportant. Thus the Filipino healers described
above pay little attention to the individual. Western
medicine has been criticised for giving too little attention
to the patient and too much to the disease, dealing with
individuals rapidly and mechanically. However, compared with
the GP's average consultation time of six minutes[4], the
Filipinos spend on average less than one minute per patient!
The reason for this is that they locate the cause of the
affliction as an invasion of the individual and try to
exorcize it or cut it out. Their treatment attacks the witch
and is not concerned with the individuals who are afflicted,
except in so far as such individuals form a site for the
'disease' of witchcraft.

However, if illness is seen as caused by disharmony in the
balance of forces within the body, then the individual
becomes all important. Treatment concentrates upon
returning the individual to his normal balanced state. Such
treatment stresses 'the whole person' and is individualistic. This is normally seen as the typical stance of
alternative medicine, giving time and care, but as I have
pointed out above, some alternative practices give little
time and little care. Finally, if illness is seen as a
resultant of environmental pressures, the individual once
again fades out of the picture and the emphasis is placed
upon changing the environment, natural or social regardless
of the individual.

With this more complex picture, we can look once again at
the question of successful healing practice. For those
healers who believe illness is a result of invaders, success
is the ousting of those invaders. For those healers who
believe illness is a disharmony within an individual,
success is the restoration of harmony. Finally, for those

healers who see illness as a resultant of environmental disturbance, success is the restoration or creation of environmental harmony. It is important to note here that orthodox medicine and unorthodox healers can be found in each of these categories. The simplistic notion of orthodox medicine as only existing in the first category is wrong just as the simplistic notion of healers only existing in the second category is equally wrong[5]. This point will be raised again later in the book and looked at in more detail.

For the moment let us turn away from healers and look at patients. It is all very well to look at healers' notions of success but it is after all the patient who is ill. Healers may well claim success when their patients do not agree. This is as true of unorthodox as conventional medicine; the old surgical joke 'the operation was successful but the patient died' is parallelled by the healer who saw death as the ultimate healing. I am not convinced the relatives of the dead person would necessarily agree with either of them. There is a clear division between the patient's criteria of success and the healer's. All healers have open to them, ultimately, only three criteria by which they can judge their success (see Lewis, 1953):

(1) the patient's feelings;
(2) manifest signs of improvement on the part of the patient;
(3) mysterious signs detected by special instruments or procedures of divination which can range from x-ray machines to the casting of knucklebones on the floor.

Of these criteria the first two are the most important to the patient in determining whether the therapy has worked. He may be shown x-ray plates or have the knucklebones interpreted but in both cases he has to accept the healer's word. For the healer, however, the last category may be more important; it is no good the patient saying he is feeling better if the doctor has irrefutable evidence of leukaemia. For the patient success is the feeling of being well and the alleviation or removal of symptoms. For the healer success is always the eradication of the cause of the affliction whether he locates the cause in invaders, imbalance in the individual or disharmony in the environment. It is thus perfectly possible for the healer to claim a success when the patient perceives a failure as was pointed out above. It is also possible, as the Baguio doctor suggested, for the patient to perceive a success when a healer sees a failure.

'Are the methods used effective?' and 'Are people healed?' cannot be given simple answers. Nor can they be given answers solely by examining Filipino healers or even all unorthodox healers. Once we ask what do we mean by healed, what do we mean by effective, we have to ask the same questions of conventional medicine. The answer we get depends on who we ask and what they see as the cause of illness. For the patient who wants relief from his symptoms and a feeling of well-being, the criteria are simple. For

the healer, orthodox or unorthodox, they are more complex,
resting as they do on his notions of the causes of illness.
For the moment the question must be held in abeyance. To
begin to struggle towards an answer we are going to have to
look at many more healers and raise questions about how some
treatments work, what are scientific criteria of success,
what is the relationship between conventional and
unconventional medicine and finally what is an individual.
(For the three sets of ideas about the causes of illness
carry within them ideas of what it means to be a person.)
This will be the theme of the rest of this book.

NOTES

(1)   'Folk Tradition in Filipino Student Cultures: A Study
      of Cebuano Preternatural Beliefs'. Sillimum Journal.
      vol. 2, no. 4 (1977) reported in the (Manila) Evening
      Post. Also see F.R. Demetrio, Dictionary of Philippine
      Folk Beliefs and Customs (Xavier University, Cagayan de
      Oro City, 1970, Library of Congress Card No. 78-
      150504).
(2)   For an account of such healers which gives a breakdown
      of the cases they deal with see Lieban (1965, 1966,
      1967).
(3)   R.G. Tajon, Alex Orbito, Exponent of Spiritual Therapy
      (World Mission Society, P.O. Box 4388, Manila,
      Philippines). Sold to me on my first visit for 80 pesos
      (about 5 pounds - an enormous sum in Filipino terms).
          The quotations about and from Alex Orbito are taken
      from this source. The description of other healers, the
      Union Esperitista and the quotations by a Belgian and a
      Baguio doctor later in the chapter are drawn from a
      series of Filipino newspaper articles most of which
      were by Vic Villafranca. These were lent to me as a
      series of cuttings by a friend and were undated. I have
      photocopies of them.
(4)   See Cartwright and O'Brien (1978) who report an average
      consultation time of just over 6 minutes for patients
      in social class I and less than 5 minutes for those in
      social class V.
(5)   This distinction underlies Fabrega and Silver's (1973)
      comparison of folk and western medicine and is a
      commonplace of interpretations of unorthodox healing by
      British healers, e.g. see the evidence presented to the
      Royal Commission on the NHS by the Healing Research
      Trust.

2 Spiritualism

The psychic surgeons of the Philippines belong to a
spiritualist movement. So too do the people and groups
described in this chapter. However, once you read the
descriptions of the practices of the English spiritualists
given below you will soon become aware that the term
'spiritualists' can cover a wide variety of practices and
theories and that more than physical distance separates the
Filipino psychic surgeons from Harry Edwards and White Eagle
Lodge. Despite the obvious differences, however, it is a
similarity that is the concern of this chapter. This
similarity is that both in the Philippines and in England
spiritualist healers have been profoundly influenced by
conventional medicine. An examination of this influence will
be used to raise the general question of the relationship of
unconventional to conventional medicine.

HARRY EDWARDS

In 1976, when I was doing my research into spiritualist
healing, the central figure amongst spiritualist healers was
Harry Edwards. Born in Holloway in 1893, he was a printer
like his father until 1935, when, after attending a service
at a spiritualist church in Ilford, he began part time
healing, an activity that eventually dominated his life. By
1955, largely through his efforts, 'The National Federation
of Spiritual Healers' was formed, an organisation that now
has over 5,000 members. When I met him[1] he was running,
with the aid of Ray and Joan Branch, the 'Harry Edwards
Spiritual Healing Centre' at Burrows Lea. This was a large
stone house sited at Shere, near Guildford, in the Surrey
countryside. There he carried out two kinds of healing
practice: contact healing and absent healing.

Contact healing

To observe contact healing I travelled on the Southern
Region train from South London to Guildford. Standing
outside Guildford Station I suddenly began to wonder how I'd
recognise the car which was to take me to the sanctuary. The
letter, from Harry Edwards, had just said a car meets the
London train.

I need not have worried, the driver held up a placard
announcing the sanctuary. I got in the back with three
ladies, two middle-aged, one young. For them, as for me, it
was their first visit. The man sitting in the front beside
the driver said it was his sixty-fourth visit. He'd come
from California. While we were chatting, the car had left
Guildford and was passing through lush countryside along a
main road which twisted and turned through several villages.
We turned off the main road and went up a steep hill along a
narrow road which was banked on either side and overhung
with trees. Finally we went through a gap in the bank and
along a gravel drive to pull into a gravel courtyard in
front of a large stone house. The house had obviously been
built in the twenties or thirties in the 'Elizabethan
Cotswold' style, a semi-fortified small manor house. The
main entrance, marked by a step and a large oak door, faced
us. To our left and behind us were the trees and shrubs
through which the drive had snaked. To our right was a wing
of the house and at the junction of that wing and the main
edifice there was a door opening and standing outside that
door was a middle aged lady with a clipboard.

We went over to her and she checked off our names on a
list as she welcomed us. Inside the door, a younger lady
dressed in a white coat (who I later found to be Joan
Branch) also welcomed us and checked off our names while
directing us to the cloakrooms if we needed them. The room
we had entered was really a corridor paved with tiles and
with glass walls to our left. It was in fact like a narrow
conservatory and contained a hotch-potch collection of
plants, busts, plaques, pictures and even a boar's head.

After relieving ourselves in the cloakroom we were guided
into the room on our right which constituted most of the
space in the wing. As people entered Joan Branch wished them
good afternoon, invited them to take a seat and asked for
their (appointment) card (which gave their name.)

The room was the setting for the contact healing. It
looked and felt like a protestant chapel and those in it
awaiting the healer whispered to each other just as
churchgoers do before a service. The focal point of the room
was a small alcove which contained a dark refectory table
above which was hung on the wall a wooden cross in a circle.
Directly in front of the alcove was a chair in dark wood
with rounded armrests flanked by rushwork seats. In front of
the chair was a long low stool with a tapestry cushion. The
feeling of being in a chapel was heightened by the pew-like
arrangement of the seats for the visitors and the presence
of a lectern, an offertory plate and some naive prints
tucked away at the back of the room. The only other item of
decoration in the room was a bust of Harry Edwards, in
bronze, set off in one corner.

Joan Branch left the room after we had been sitting for
five or ten minutes, announcing, 'We'll start now.'
Everyone stopped talking and looked expectantly at the door.

Through the door came Harry Edwards accompanied by Joan and Ray Branch all of them dressed in white coats. Harry Edwards had the build and the presence of the elderly Winston Churchill. After wishing everyone good afternoon he sat in the central chair with Joan Branch on his right and Ray Branch on his left. Everyone then prayed, in silence, for a short time before the healing session began.

The session was organised and orchestrated by Joan Branch who signalled each person to come up and sit on the tapestry stool, gave out pamphlets when asked to by Harry Edwards and informed him of any knowledge about the affliction of the patient as he or she approached the stool. She also, along with her husband, helped Harry Edwards with some of the patients. I have selected three examples from my field notes that illustrate the process:

Example 1. The man from California. A tall man in his early sixties with a relaxed American style about him. He left his seat after a signal from Joan Branch, shook hands with Harry Edwards and sat on the stool.

Words	Actions
HARRY EDWARDS: How are things now?	He holds the hand of the Californian and feels his neck, keeping his eyes closed.
Is it painful?	Ray Branch stands behind the man with one hand on his right shoulder and the other on the back of his neck.
This has less consistency than before.	
CALIFORNIAN: It's smaller.	
HARRY EDWARDS: Lighter. You respond very quickly, don't you? Feel how soft it is. What else is wrong?	
JOAN BRANCH: His hip	Harry Edwards moves the man's head back and forward, then round, then turns it. The Californian is holding his back rigid.
CALIFORNIAN: It's arthritis.	
HARRY EDWARDS: Today it's not too bad.	Harry Edwards and Ray Branch rock the man backward and forward on the stool.
That's all right	Harry Edwards takes the man's hand again.
CALIFORNIAN: Ever since you started it's been coming back slowly.	
HARRY EDWARDS: Do you help yourself as much as you help other people?	
CALIFORNIAN: Get most help from you.	
HARRY EDWARDS: We're always here.	Harry Edwards looks him in the eye and smiles.

24

Example 2. A young woman in her mid twenties looking withdrawn and closed in upon herself, dressed in conventional clothes. She goes and sits on the stool.

Words	Actions
	Harry Edwards holds her hand and then places a hand on her breast.
WOMAN: I had surgery two years ago.	
HARRY EDWARDS: No other secondaries?	Harry Edwards takes her hand and releases it.
WOMAN: I've got cancer of the liver.	Harry Edwards takes her hand again.
HARRY EDWARDS: It's all away from you at the breasts.	Harry Edwards places a hand on her abdomen through a gap in her dress and starts massaging it.
WOMAN: I'm on drugs, it doesn't seem to be responding.	
HARRY EDWARDS: Do the injections upset you?	
WOMAN: I hate them but they don't make me feel ill.	Harry Edwards, still massaging her abdomen asks Joan Branch to help him. The woman has her eyes closed.
HARRY EDWARDS: Are you eating well?	
WOMAN: Eating well, feeling well.	
HARRY EDWARDS: On a diet?	
WOMAN: No.	
HARRY EDWARDS: No pain?	
WOMAN: No.	
HARRY EDWARDS: We'd like you to come in for a special healing treatment for this trouble. What you'll be getting is a whole course. There's a small questionnaire - fill it in and from that time there will be special intercession. (To Joan Branch.) Getting soft now, Joan, going down. Rest of the tummy swells up - whether that's fluid or not...? (To woman.) Feel that, it's gone down.	He is still massaging her abdomen.
WOMAN: Yes.	
HARRY EDWARDS: Don't worry about it, be convinced you will get better.	

25

WOMAN: I am convinced

HARRY EDWARDS: It's clear
you're receptive, clear
you're going to be helped

Joan Branch gets the
questionnaire from a
drawer in the refectory
table and gives it to the
woman.

WOMAN: Am I to come
back?

HARRY EDWARDS: We do
hold special days or you
can make special
arrangements for an
appointment.

The woman stands up and
Ray Branch shows her out
through a door at the back
of the room.

Example 3. A middle aged lady and her husband. The husband
and the lady are both dressed in suits, having dressed
formally for the trip and for the occasion.

Because the husband comes up with his wife there is some
rearrangement of position. The husband is seated in the
chair to Harry Edwards's right and Joan Branch moves into
the chair on his left.

Words	Actions
HARRY EDWARDS: Where do you get the arthritis?	Harry Edwards holds her hand.
WOMAN: In the back.	Ray Branch holds her back.
HARRY EDWARDS: Do you get pain in the spine?	Harry Edwards and Ray Branch rock her back and forth on the stool.
WOMAN: It's shrunk.	
HARRY EDWARDS: Collapsed, not shrunk, got fast, got fused. No cementing there now. Let's look at the top of you, looser, it's as simple as that, no, let the head go right back. I shan't hurt you. Take it right back now.	Harry Edwards is moving her head and back and Ray Branch is moving her arm like a slow piston.
Let it swing, don't move your body, take it up and down, bend the elbow, let it fall. (To husband.) Are you the husband? The back of the spine yielded very nicely, neck as well. Main thing to maintain the healing is the movement. We're opening them and having got them open keep them open. Movement is the enemy of arthritis.	Harry Edwards takes over the arm.

26

(To woman.) Do this every day and if you find your neck is tight, move it and keep it moving, don't put up with it. Better shoulder?

WOMAN: I'm left handed and use this one.

Harry Edwards moves her left arm like a slow piston.

HARRY EDWARDS: Easy?

WOMAN: A bit.

HARRY EDWARDS (jokingly): Only a bit?

WOMAN: It is easier.

At this stage everyone in the room is looking on in fascination, sitting forward in their chairs. Joan Branch starts looking closely at the woman's left forearm.

HARRY EDWARDS (to Joan Branch): Stiff muscle.

WOMAN: I put it in a plaster cast each night.

HARRY EDWARDS: That's the medical way - hold it tight so it doesn't hurt. Our purpose is to get it loose. Personally I wouldn't use it again - warmth, heat, massage, bathing in hot water - all these things are good.

Harry Edwards takes her hand.

Strangely enough your little finger was the bad one. That's gone very well, gone beautifully. Do it yourself now. Are your legs bad?

He rubs the finger back and forward.

WOMAN: My feet are bad.

HARRY EDWARDS: Can I have a foot up here?

Woman takes off her shoe and puts the right foot, still in her nylon stocking, on Harry Edwards's knee.

WOMAN: Had operations on both feet, this was the recent one.

HARRY EDWARDS: I shan't hurt you. What did they do?

Harry Edwards rotates foot.

WOMAN: The toe was underneath, they brought it up but it's gone under again.

JOAN BRANCH: Was it further out?

27

HARRY EDWARDS: I shan't hurt you. Let them come up, let them come over - that's got them all loose. It would help if you walk on your toes each day. Buy one of those Scholl contraptions. They've made a good job of that. Let's look at the other one.

Harry Edwards manipulates her toes.

WOMAN: The toe gets painful on the bottom when I'm walking.

Woman raises her other foot.

HARRY EDWARDS: Shan't hurt you. Let it go round on that point, right, next one. See (Joan Branch). Put tape on it, it will come round.

Harry Edwards manipulates her toes.

He gets Joan Branch to move it by guiding her fingers.

WOMAN: Thank you very much Mr Edwards.

JOAN BRANCH: (to Harry Edwards): Diabetes.

HARRY EDWARDS: Is your sight all right?

WOMAN: I've got cataracts on both eyes.

HARRY EDWARDS: Not so bad, healing of this does take time. It's a case of altering function, not like a joint. Mrs Branch is going to take you over there to see to your eyes.

Edwards holds abdomen.

Joan Branch gets a leaflet on arthritis from the drawer, gives it to Harry Edwards who gives it to the woman.

(To husband) Massage is good. Can you go over there?

The couple go off with Joan Branch to the back of the room.

The explanation of the healing practice I had just observed was given by Harry Edwards and Mr and Mrs Branch in these terms:

HARRY EDWARDS: You see healing is a gift. You don't learn it by going on a course of study. It is largely dependent on a person's character, aptitude and...on his genetic abilities...Healers are invariably those who are generous in their nature, people who will support causes and fight for causes without getting a result or a reward. They must have an

innate   yearning to help those who seek, they have
compassion. They are the   people who you find
possess the gift of healing...The quality of the
healing in my mind depends entirely on the degree of
attunement...a healer can establish with a source of
healing. To bring about a change, a state of change in
anything, in the universe must be the result of applied,
law governed, forces. This applies to healing too. And
when a physical change takes place such as with
arthritis, the dispersal of a cataract - whatever it
might be - the result follows the application of law
governed energies or forces to make the chemical change.
To operate that there must be an intelligence that has
the ability of getting together those energies in their
right strength and so forth in order to create the
molecules of energy that are directed to the patient to
make the necessary change in the physical state - to the
shoulder or the eyes or whatever it might be. And as
that intelligence is not human, because no human mind
has this ability, it does prove in my mind, the
existence of another realm of intelligence, which we
call the spirit world. Animating all this is the divine
intention. I think healing is God's gift to all his
people, irrespective of age or colour or religion. And
it is that source of healing, where these intelligences
are, that we are able to get in contact with...through
meditation and...attunement...in order for healing to
take place. In other words, I've not done any healing
this afternoon. It's all taken place through me, it's
not been me.
Healing is much easier today. Now I've already said,
whether you believe it or not, that in order to give a
result you must be applying a given therapy. That's the
result of wisdom and knowledge. If, as the years have
gone by, those whom I call our spirit doctors, if they
have been able to acquire greater knowledge...then
they've got a greater knowledge and greater powers of
diagnosis. They know more about the physical laws and
the spirit laws that govern the universe, and they're
able to give more than they did then. Also they may be
accustomed to using people like me better. Maybe I'm a
better instrument[2].

SELF: How do you diagnose?
JOAN BRANCH: One's guided by impressions. We don't diagnose
    as such.
SELF: Impression?
JOAN BRANCH: Just a thought that's given to you. Impressions
    come from the spirit. Impression and the directive comes
    before you go to the part concerned...
RAY BRANCH: You might have a patient here and you'll go
    there (he points to abdomen) and just scan across it
    (moves his hand). Now you'll get an impression there's
    something not quite as it should be. This might be the
    result of some abdominal surgery.
JOAN BRANCH: It is a complete question of attunement and the
    experience of how to define that attunement and the

29

thoughts that one gets. We are only used as channels aren't we? Healing is really the simplest thing in the world because we do not do it[3].

Absent healing

Absent healing or distance healing as it is called by some healers formed the major part of the activities at Burrows Lea. Directly opposite the front door is a large office which deals with the daily influx of letters. Harry Edwards estimated they received ten thousand letters a week and even allowing for some exaggeration there is no doubt that the flow of requests, petitions, pleas and thanks was very large. It would appear, from Harry Edwards's own account that absent healing as a major part of his work was forced upon him by his own success:

> In the years preceding the last war and during the first war years, an ever increasing number of sick people wrote to me for absent healing or came to my home for personal treatment...
> The number of sufferers who came in person became so great that our front room and sanctuary could not accommodate them all and queues formed outside in the street...I was therefore compelled to institute a system of appointments for personal healing and leave some evenings free for absent healing.
> The successful and high percentage of recoveries taking place through absent healing showed me this should be my major concern[4].

The actual process of absent healing is described in a pamphlet distributed by the sanctuary:

> All spiritual healing is a gradual process. Sensational or 'miracle' healings do take place on occasion, but they are an exception to the general rule.
> Absent healing intercessions commence from the time the necessary request is made to the healer, usually by way of a letter, which gives the healer a mind picture of the patient's needs.
> Every healing request receives individual attention, and each patient is interceded for individually. Thus, every letter is answered personally...
> For Absent Healing to be conducted with purpose and direction, the healers depend upon the information you are able to give them, thus:
> 1. Weekly letters are of the utmost importance in monitoring the continuity of the healing purpose...
> There are not set times for patients to link up in thought with the healing intercessions. We believe that those with whom we are in attunement on behalf of patients, work unceasingly to bring about all possible betterment.
> ...with chronic complaints, the first task of the

spirit doctors is to stay the progress of the
disease, thus preventing any further deterior-
ation[5].

I was fortunate enough to be given access to some of these
letters during my visit with the proviso that I did not take
the letters out of the sanctuary or break their
confidentiality. Thus I was given, for a morning only, two
files labelled 'special file' and 'cancer file'. The special
file contained letters sent to the sanctuary and selected
out by Harry Edwards and his close associates as being from
patients who had 'done well'. The term 'done well' was Harry
Edwards's phrase and when I used the term 'cure' he
corrected me and insisted on 'done well'. The file was a
twelve month running file, the first letter dated 29 October
1975 and the last 12 October 1976. There were in total fifty
three letters referring to seventy six individuals. The
cancer file was also a twelve month running file and
contained all letters written in the past year which
referred to cancer. The sanctuary was running a special
study of cancer which involved monitoring all cancer
clients:

Seventeen years ago I was quite sure that the cause
of cancer was not organic, that it was
psychosomatic...I've lately had, in the last few
years, an opportunity to develop it...
We started off with eight cases of terminal cancer
- we got the people to lose their fear of it, to talk
about it. We got them to look forward to getting
better, not to have the dread of cancer. They're
going to get better from it. We got them to do half
an hour's meditation a day. And we got them to come
to a healing once a week, once a month, whatever it
was. The result was that after two years fifty per
cent were still alive and radiant in health. We lost
four, and so I said, 'If we can do that that way I'm
going to try and do it by absent healing.' I have
great faith in absent healing. So last September we
started and we asked for people who knew they had
cancer to come in. These are some of the cases we are
now dealing with.
We've got five hundred cases now of cancers of all
kinds. Some are not serious, but most of them are
serious. They answer a questionnaire in which they
give us the medical testimony as to their trouble,
name of their hospital, name of their doctor, what
the doctors say, that is all we can go on. Then we
have them and we get them to do the same things. Half
an hour's meditation a day, we supply them with
instructions how to do it. We give them also the
inspiration to look forward to getting better. The
whole treatment is designed with that outlook, and
they write in once a week, these files are all their
letters...Now and again we get a whole afternoon of
cancer patients, and so we do what we are doing now:
we get them to look forward, have no fear and so
on[2].

31

Many of the letters in the cancer file were harrowing and depressing, impassioned pleas for help from a relative or friend of the person who was afflicted[6]. The special file, as one would expect, made happier reading. These are specially selected to be used in the pamphlets and books of the sanctuary as examples of healing. The largest number of letters in the special file report a healing. This is most often a simple statement that their affliction is 'cured' or 'healed' but is occasionally a detailed testimonial such as that given by a woman about her brother-in-law who had a leg amputated and then:

> He refused to have his other leg off and discharged himself from the hospital. His condition was such that he was delirious and rambling most of the time, his weight had dropped to four stone and he was obviously dying. After writing to you he immediately started to recover and after three months he was able to get about in a wheelchair and put weight on...he is now in the best of health and drives around in an invalid car.

Then there are those who report that the sick person is now functioning or has managed to return to work, e.g. 'Without your help I would be in a hospital bed...I am today able to sit on top of a hill in Sussex.' Others report improvement, e.g. 'Although the doctors told us they could do nothing for my son's sight - no hope - since coming to Burrows Lea for contact healing and absent healing - although there is very slow progress there is progress.' Finally, there are those who have managed to avoid a dreaded operation or who say they are no longer centred on their illness or just generally feel better or have not got worse[7].

WHITE EAGLE LODGE

Unlike the spiritual healing sanctuary of Harry Edwards, which looks like many similar large houses in the area, White Eagle Lodge stands apart from the surrounding countryside: the thatched cottages and sunken lanes of Hampshire. In the midst of this, sitting on top of a small rise with magnificent views over the surrounding countryside, glaring white against the sky and fields and looking like an observatory, is White Eagle Lodge. A domed building with a neoclassical entrance, stretching two thirds of its height, surmounted by stylized, elongated, bronze wings.

Inside there is a sign 'Please preserve the silence' and taped music of the 'pop classic' variety. Once out of the entrance foyer you step under the dome. Except for the facing wall the walls curve round the sides of the dome, covered to above head height by blue curtains. The facing wall consists of a small stage with four central steps leading up to it, the steps flanked by white scroll ironwork balustrades. At the top of the steps there is an altar covered in a yellow cloth which is lit from above. Hanging over the altar is a large 'diamond' which is spot lighted. Behind the altar there is a cream drapery hanging down from the ceiling in front of yellow walls. Either side of the altar there are matching floral displays. On the stage on both sides of the steps are a tapestry chair and lectern fronted with matching tapestry. The walls immediately at the side of the stage do not have the blue curtain that stretches around the rest of the 'room' but instead go clear to the ceiling and have eight large speakers mounted on them (four on each side). Below the speakers there are hymn boards and below them two ornately backed black chairs. The floor of the body of the 'hall' is green as are the modern chairs ranked on it facing the altar. The stage is carpeted in russet and the dome is black. Around the circumference of the bottom of the dome, set against a white background, are large gold symbols.

The overall effect on me, in spite of the symbolism, was not one of mysticism. It was rather as though the front parlour of a 'respectable' working class home had been writ large and redesigned so that everyone could come for tea.

The Lodge is called White Eagle Lodge after the spirit that guides the members of the Lodge:

> White Eagle is the name by which we know a very wise and loving soul who has guided the work of the Lodge from the spirit world for many years.
> He speaks through Grace Cooke, words of great love and wisdom...
> We believe that White Eagle has also had an important incarnation in France where the symbol of the six pointed star was used by the particular Brotherhood he served. In Greece, as well as in Egypt, he was a teacher and philosopher. As a North American Indian, he lived to a great age; and according to his own story was a chief among the six tribes of the Iroquois...
> His usual personality is of the old American Indian Chieftain, but he is also familiar to many of his friends as a Tibetan, an Egyptian Priest Pharaoh, a humble brother in an obscure order, and an alchemist of the Middle Ages. Whatever bodies and personalities have been his in the past, he remains, to us, dear old White Eagle[8].
> The method of healing practised at the White Eagle Lodge is a unique and powerful method involving co-operation with the angels of healing. The angels work with the healers to direct the healing in the form of colour rays which bring to the patient's soul the qualities it needs. They strengthen his spirit which then works gradually to bring all the bodies into harmony and health. These rays are projected to the patients through the soul power of the healers and the magical assistance of the angels, without which

healing could not take place. The following colour rays are used:

1. Red, from the deepest to the very palest rose pink.
2. Gold, from palest sunlight to rich deep orange.
3. Green, especially a bright fresh spring green and also a golden green, like sunlight through the green leaves of spring.
4. Blue, from palest sky blue to rich deep delphinium or madonna blue.
5. Violet, ranging from palest amethyst to the colour of deep rich violets.
6. The pearl or Christ Light ray - in which is contained all the other colours.

These colours, seen clairvoyantly, are bright and translucent, like sunlight shining through a very beautiful stained glass window. Each colour brings a particular quality to fill some lack in the soul, and is chosen accordingly. They are usually directed to the psychic centres in the etheric body which through the ductless glands and nerve centres are linked with different physical organs. Remember that the healer aims to reach and heal the basic cause of the trouble deep within the soul-body.

Healing power works gently. Since most disease starts in the soul-body and may have taken years to build up and show in the physical body, it is not surprising that it may be some weeks, months, or even years before the effects of the healing are felt upon the physical body. The fact that no change is visible in the physical condition does not mean that the healing is proving ineffective. Remember, it is working first on the soul-body, and often the first sign of the healing which is taking place will be a feeling of inner peace, of being able to cope with life. Gradually this will reach the physical body, the atoms of which will be commanded by the Divine Will in the healer and patient to return to harmony so that well-being, and good health will result.

The colour ray healing we give at the White Eagle Lodge is of two types:

Contact Healing: As the name implies, this involves direct contact between healer and patient. It usually takes place as part of a Healing Service at the Lodge, in which each patient receives individual treatment from one of our trained healers.

Absent Healing: Since it is the soul-body which is being treated, and this lies beyond the confines of physical law, the rays can be sent to the patient from a distance. To do this, groups of trained healers sit together regularly at the Lodges, or as part of a Lone Healing group. Patients are told how to co-operate by tuning in to these rays before going to sleep at night. Each group of healers is under the leadership of one who is directly linked with the

Star Brotherhood in the invisible world. The power and effectiveness of the healing depends entirely on this magical link.

That this healing in either form is effective is beyond all doubt. We have had many 'miracle' cures, as well as very many less spectacular but just as impressive, a quiet and gradual healing taking place over the months. There can be few things more rewarding than to see the progress of patients from sickness to health and happiness. And all who take part as healers testify to the blessing and joy their service brings to their lives[9].

ORTHODOX MEDICINE AND HEALING

For many centuries there was no 'orthodox' medicine. Healing was conducted by individuals using a variety of methods based on even more various theories of illness. What we now consider to be the orthodox was just one amongst a variety of healing methods and theories. If there was an orthodoxy in healing it was provided by the Church: the registrars of holy shrines 'consistently emphasized the superiority of sacred over profane healing. It was often said to be foolish and rash to seek the help of human doctors in the first place' (Finucane, 1977, p.64). When the Church's dominance over life began to decline at the time of the Reformation so too did its dominance over healing. This is not to say that religious healing declined. It did not. Rather it was no longer possible for the Church to claim religious healing as the orthodox method and others as alternatives.

With the decline of the Church as the arbiter of acceptable healing practice a 'free for all' developed with all the various modes of healing claiming legitimacy for their methods. This anarchic situation lasted until the nineteenth century when with Pasteur's work a new orthodoxy emerged triumphant. The emergence of this new orthodoxy, modern medicine, is usually presented as a process of progress - the inevitable triumph of truth over error, of science over ignorance and of effective medicine over quackery. The truth is as usual more complex than this simplistic view of history suggests. Orthodox medicine became the orthodoxy by defeating some rival theories of illness and incorporating others, and these defeats and incorporations had more to do with the relevant power positions of the competing parties than any ideas of truth, science and effectiveness. To illustrate this point let us look first at what we now know as orthodox medicine in operation in the seventeenth century, when it was just one theory - allopathy - amongst many. Allopathy, which is today the orthodox, saw the cause of illness as the invasion of the body by toxic materials. Therapy therefore consisted of the purging of these toxic materials out of the body by the use of enemas and bleeding. Fundamental to the theory and practice of allopathy, then as now, was a concentration upon disease symptoms and an attempt to reduce the symptoms of a disease. Then, as now, it was the sick individual in isolation from his environment who was the concern of the doctor. Also, then as now, doctors claimed that they were acting scientifically.

An alternative theory of disease and an alternative therapy was available to men in the seventeenth century, namely astrology. This too claimed scientific validity; and provided both an explanation for illness and therapeutic practices[10]. The success of allopathy and the decline of astrology as an explanation and treatment of illness was not due to any greater efficacy on the part of allopathy. Allopathy, with its purges and leeches, was as likely to kill as to cure in this period. Nor was its success due to allopathy's greater scientific validity. The claim to be scientific was probably more justified for astrology than allopathy. Its success was due to two factors: better organisation and a congruence between its theories and those of the elite. Allopathy had better organisation because the core[11] members of the medical profession formed a small social group in London, a group in close contact with the political elite. Although there were astrologers acting for the elite they did not form a coherent group. Perhaps, more important for the triumph of allopathy was the shift in the world view of the elite which took place in this period[12]: astrology was integrated into the old world view, allopathy to the new. Astrology had a view of the universe that saw man as but part of a 'great chain of being' living in harmony with nature: the chain stretched from inanimate rocks through animals and man to the angels, saints and finally God. Astrology saw illness as being a result of disharmony and therapy as the restoration of harmony. Its practice was open to all men who would undertake the requisite study. In contrast allopathy adopted the new individualistic, rationalistic view of the universe with the emphasis upon the individual and upon the domination of nature - the view that the ruling class increasingly adopted as their own. Thus by the turn of the century allopathic medicine was triumphant and astrology discredited amongst the elite.

However, the defeat of astrology did not mean that allopathy reigned alone as the only mode of explanation of illness. The eighteenth and nineteenth centuries saw a proliferation of theories some of which survive today as alternative medicine. One theory in particular presented a very real challenge to allopathy, that of homoeopathy. Developed in 1796 by a German physician, Hahnemann, homoeopathy argued that it was not the invasion of toxic forces that caused illness but rather the weakness of the 'life force' in the patient. Hahnemann argued that if illness was to be explained by the invasion of toxic forces then why should some die and some live during an epidemic: surely there must be differences in individuals which are more important than any invading forces? Therapy should concentrate not on driving out toxic invaders but on building up the life force of the individual. The way to build up this life force, believed Hahnemann, was to administer small doses of drugs to produce similar symptoms to those produced by the disease. Homoeopathy was very influential in the nineteenth century and still survives today in the practice of immunisation as well as in the homoeopathic hospitals and doctors of London.

For most doctors, however, the conflict between homoeopathy and allopathy was resolved by Pasteur's discovery of germs. Germs, they believed, were obviously the invading toxic forces allopathic physicians had pointed to for centuries: scientific investigation had proved allopathy to be correct. From that time allopathy emerged as the clear orthodoxy. So much so that it could afford to incorporate other therapies under its wing even when their theories were in complete conflict with its own. We have already seen that immunisation, a homoeopathic practice, was incorporated into orthodox medicine. Similar incorporations have continued until the present day. For example, the nineteenth century phenomena of mesmerism, which was initially rejected, was finally incorporated under a new name, hypnosis, with the proviso that when used for therapeutic purposes it should be used only by qualified medical men[13]. A more recent example is provided by acupuncture where once again orthodox medical practitioners have demanded that it only be practised by licensed practitioners, i.e. themselves[14]. In my own work I have come across similar attempts to incorporate alternative practice. The Psionic Medical Society (see Chapter 4) want to reserve radiesthesia as a diagnostic and therapeutic tool to qualified doctors and the director of a health centre (see Chapter 5) wants to bring alternative practitioners under the supervision of a qualified medical practitioner.

As this book demonstrates the dominance of allopathic, conventional, medicine has not meant the demise of alternative medical theories and therapies. When people suffer from an affliction they are not too interested in theories, they want relief. To find that relief they will use a variety of paths, which path they choose being dependent on such factors as accessibility, legitimacy and respectability (New, 1977). Nonetheless although alternative medicine and conventional medicine exist side by side there is no doubt that the predominant model is that of conventional medicine. Even in societies which have incorporated traditional healers into their medical care systems such as Tanzania (Dunlop, 1975) and China (New and New, 1975, 1977), such healers have been subject to the overview of doctors trained in orthodox medicine. While in our own society, despite critiques of conventional medicine as a system which steals the autonomy of the individual (Illich, 1974), the major mode of coping with affliction is that presented by conventional medicine. This dominance is so deep that alternative medicine can only be said to exist in the shadow of orthodox medicine. Orthodox medicine colours the practice of alternative medicine and affects its operation profoundly. It does so when alternative practitioners adopt the symbols of conventional medicine, e.g. Harry Edwards and his helpers wear white coats like doctors and Harry Edwards's guiding spirits were Lord Lister and Louis Pasteur, both prominent figures in the development of orthodox medicine. Nor is Harry Edwards alone in this practice. The cymatic practitioner we shall encounter later (Chapter 4) also wears a white coat and conducts himself when examining his patients just like a doctor on ward rounds. Chiropractors have their working offices laid out with all the symbols of a doctor, including such things as framed diplomas on the walls (Cowie and Roebuck, 1975). Even in the exotic practice of bare-hand surgery by Alex Orbito there are indications that the practice is derived from observation of western surgeons.

If orthodox medicine provides props for the alternative practitioner to appropriate this however is only a small part of its contribution. More importantly it provides services to alternative medicine. The first service it provides is to be an alternative for the alternative practitioner. When he finds a case he cannot deal with because it is outside the scope of his practice he refers the patient to orthodox medicine.Thus, throughout the world, alternative practitioners send those with serious accidental injuries on to hospital and often they send also those who would be more efficiently treated by antibiotics.Finally they also sometimes send those they consider are dying and for whom they know they can do nothing; thus it is the hospital that has a failure rather than the healer[15]. The second service it provides is to be a filter for the healer. Where conventional medicine is freely and easily available, as in Britain for example, the doctor is usually the first resort of the afflicted individual. This has several consequences for the healer. Doctors get swamped but healers are only overloaded, for the initial wave of illness breaks upon the doctor's door not the healers. This enables the healer to give more time to his patient than the doctor and many healers are aware of this[16]. It also means that the healer does not need to concern himself with diagnosis. The doctor does the diagnosis for him and he receives it secondhand, from the patient. None of the healers I studied were at all concerned with diagnosis. Even those using radiethesia, which is in essence a diagnostic rather than a therapeutic technique, in practice relied on a doctor's diagnosis rather than their own (see Chapter 4). Finally, it means that healers do not deal with crisis illnesses - with accident emergencies such as amputated hands or torn skin or such medical emergencies as fever. If people with such afflictions do by some chance present themselves to the healer, then, as was noted above, they send them off to the doctor. Rather they deal with chronic illnesses and incurable diseases, afflictions that the doctor has been unable to deal with. Therefore alternative medicine cannot be antagonistic to orthodox medicine but is rather dependent upon it for many of its symbols, and more importantly for the services orthodox medicine provides by acting as a front line in the battle against affliction.

CONCLUSION

There is no doubt that orthodox medicine has been immensely
successful in dealing with certain types of affliction.
Although historical research has demonstrated that sewers
were more important than doctors in bringing down the death
rate from all sorts of diseases[17] it is still true that in
individual cases medical intervention has been crucial.
However, this very success has presented the conventional
practitioner with problems. The majority of patients who
present themselves at his surgery do not have crisis
afflictions. They are not suffering from typhus or needing
major surgery. Yet the core of allopathic medicine consists
of therapies to deal with such crisis afflictions. Thus the
medical student is expected to learn about and recognise all
sorts of diseases the great majority of which he will never
see in his life unless he works in a major teaching
hospital.

Let us caricature conventional medicine to illustrate the
point. Such a caricature, it must be pointed out, is a major
theme in comparisons of orthodox and alternative medicine.
The concept of 'disease' dominates medical thought and
medical practice. In fact it can be argued that the core
notion in allopathy is the notion of 'disease'. A 'disease'
is a process inferred from signs and symptoms observed over
time. It is an abstract entity which is presumed not to be
tied to any particular culture or historical time - Chinamen
can get measles as easily as Englishman and Victorians might
die of cholera as easily as the present day inhabitants of
Calcutta. It is important to realise that 'disease' is an
abstract concept, not an object - you cannot look at a
disease under a microscope although you may be able to look
at one of the causes of it. It is an analytic category which
groups together certain signs and symptoms. Nowadays the
notion of disease dominates conventional medicine: 'In
English, "medicine" can be given the traditional meaning of
the art of healing...or medicine can be given the meaning it
has come to have now, that is the study of the diagnosis,
treatment and prevention of disease' argues Lewis (1975,
p.147) who goes on to suggest that this distinction has
implications for the social relationship involved in the
therapeutic process: 'The traditional sense, the art of
healing, implies that medicine is concerned with people or
patients, with conditions of man; while the modern sense,
study and control of disease, implies rather study of a
thing, disease.' A point echoed by Mathers (1970, p.9) who
says 'to treat a disease means to attack, destroy or inhibit
it in some way. To treat a patient on the other hand, means
to foster, nurture or care for his capacity for living.'

So if orthodox medicine is concerned with diseases rather
than people then its practitioners will be concerned more
with things than people. It will treat the patient not as an
individual but as a site for a disease,[18] and will
therefore expect the patient to be passive (which is what
the word 'patient' means) providing information to the

39

physician and allowing a physical assault upon his body with knives, namely surgery.

Now this, as I pointed out, is a caricature. Nonetheless there is no doubt that the central aspects of allopathic theory and practice present just such a picture. However such therapeutic practices as surgery, which treats the patient as an object, a site for a disease, are only suitable for some forms of affliction and those forms are becoming less and less of a problem with increasing public health, increasing immunisation and increasing medical success. The problems now are chronic and incurable diseases - arthritis, coronaries, cancer - the so-called 'diseases of affluence' and mental diseases especially depression. For these diseases surgery and drugs provide only partial remedies. They also require a different form of social relationship. The doctor cannot intervene dramatically and produce a cure but has to engage in a long term social relationship with his patient which makes it extremely difficult to treat him or her as an object passive to his will.

One response is to try and ignore the problem; to continue treating such patients as though they had crisis afflictions. Thus the doctor gives the patient with mental illness tranquillisers and, until recently, continues dosing on repeat prescriptions. Such a response is in line with his medical training. It also helps him resolve his anxieties in a situation where he is pressed for time. Presented with a patient whose illness he cannot easily classify or treat, he prescribes. He prescribes because it reassures the patient and the doctor that action is being taken[19]. In a situation of uncertainty the doctor is happier doing something rather than nothing. This is exactly the manner in which Malinowski (1954) described magical acts amongst islanders in the Pacific: the individual faced with uncertainty feels he must act and he acts with greater precision than normal (Comaroff, 1976).

Another response is to modify the practice. Many doctors are taking this course. They are moving from a position where they are the active agent acting upon a passive patient to one where both they and the patient are neutral participants in a healing process[20]. The hospice movement and the growth of pain clinics are good examples of this type of change. Interestingly doctors who employ this response, just like Harry Edwards, reject notions of cure and use such terms as more or less successful. Some are even incorporating healers into their practice by referring patients to them.

There is thus a conflict in conventional medicine at present. On the one hand there is a long history of a theory and practice of medicine that emphasizes treatment of disease without regard to its context and treatment of the patient in an individual consultation - a theory and history enshrined in medical training and supported by a record of success. On the other hand there is increasingly an awareness that today most patients do not suffer from crisis diseases but have chronic long-term complaints. For these patients a mode of therapy that concentrates upon them as individuals in their social context seems to offer the best chance of success. However, to adopt such a mode is to return to the view of the world which sees man as part of a wider context, which is, in the eyes of many doctors, a return to the magical, astrological view of the universe. Incidentally it is this same difficulty which makes many doctors resistant to the finding of psychosomatic research in medicine. The dominant model is oriented to treating the individual and explaining diseases in terms of material forces that can be observed in the laboratory in a determinate manner. Social forces are not material (although they have material effects), they are not deterministic but probabilistic in operation, and the emphasis in explanation is not on the individual but on the social group. Healers, of course, are much readier to adopt this mode of explanation with its stress on immaterial forces and its emphasis on interpersonal relations. Doctors are thus ambivalent about the therapies used in alternative medicine. Some are profoundly antagonistic, dismissing it all as quackery[21], whereas others are only too happy to espouse the alternative 'cause'[22].

Healers have no such ambivalent attitude towards orthodox medicine. Most accept it as an essential part of their practice, and admit their dependence upon it in certain areas (as outlined earlier). What most healers want is not the abolition of orthodox medicine but its recognition of their contribution to the relief of affliction[23].

NOTES

(1) In December 1976. He died the morning after my inter-
    view.
(2) Quoted verbatim from a tape-recording of an interview
    with Harry Edwards.
(3) Quoted verbatim from a tape-recording of an interview
    with Mr and Mrs Branch.
(4) Edwards (1968), p.85.
(5) From 'Notes on Absent healing', a pamphlet of the
    Sanctuary.

41

(6)

Afflicted Person's Relationship to Letter Writer

	'Cancer file' (n-98)*	'Special file' (n=76)
Self	12	29
Parent	5	2
Son or daughter	9	9
Sibling	8	1
Spouse	18	20
In-law	12	3
Friend	13	3
Other	5	6
Unspecified	24	3

It was not possible to analyse all the cancer letters in the short time available to me so three months – February, November and December – were chosen to give a spread throughout the year. The information in all the letters was sparse, e.g. of the 76 letters in the 'special file' 13 did not specify the affliction at all and of the 98 letters in the 'cancer file' 3 did not specify the type of cancer.

   *Some of the letters in the 'cancer file' asked for help for more than one individual. So the 98 letters referred to 106 individuals.

(7)

Special File

Report of healing	23	Report of feeling better	4
Report of functioning	11	Report of not getting	
Report of improvement	7	worse	2
Report of avoiding an		(The remaining 23 are	
operation	6	requests for intercession)	

(8) From the undated pamphlet by Grace Cooke, Who is White Eagle? This quotation and the others from the literature of White Eagle Lodge are made with the kind permission of White Eagle Lodge and the White Eagle Publishing Trust of New Lands, Liss, Hampshire, who retain copyright.

(9) From the undated pamphlet Spiritual Healing, White Eagle Publishing Trust.

(10) For a detailed discussion of astrology and medicine see Wright (1979).

(11) i.e., the members of the Royal College of Physicians who held the monopoly of medical practice in London.

(12) For a detailed account of this shift see Thomas (1973)

(13) From a report of a committee of the BMA cited by Parsinnen (1979, p.116).

(14) For a description of the attempt to incorporate acupuncture see Webster (1979).

(15) This has been reported for Thai healers; see Riley and Semsri, 1974.

(16) See for example the cymatic practitioner's account of what would happen if his clinic became part of the National Health Service, p.83.
(17) See Tuckett (1976) and Clogg (1978) for a summary of the evidence that it was improvement in preventive social medicine that made and makes the most effect on life chances, not individual medicine.
(18) See Manning and Fabrega (1973) for a detailed comparison of western and traditional medicine.
(19) La Patra (1978) has a detailed account of this situation.
(20) Szasz and Hollander (1956) provide a detailed classification of the modes of relationship involved in healing.
(21) See Katz (1972) for an attack on chiropractic as quackery.
(22) For example the Scientific and Medical Network described by Eagle (1978).
(23) See the evidence given by the Scientific and Medical Network to the Royal Commission on the Health Service.

3 Christian healing

LOURDES

Journeys blur in my mind. It is impossible to remember the complete event. All that survives is a mood, an emotion, and coupled with that emotion a collection of images and impressions. The journey I took to Lourdes is like that. The emotion I retain is a feeling of pleasure, although whether this is a result of my later experiences I do not know. The images I have are of the departure lounge at Gatwick airport with people standing around chatting animatedly, of the departure ramp as the passengers clustered to go down the steps to the bus which was to take us to the airplane, and an image of a small group of young people, in their early twenties, joking with the stewardess by pretending an American accent which she saw through immediately. And, on arrival in France, of sitting on the conveyor belt at the airport waiting for luggage and then of the hospice where 'the sick' stayed - a cross between a hospital ward and my vision of a medieval monastery. And underlying all these visual images, a chatter of voices as people kept answering my question why were they going to Lourdes?

Why were they going to Lourdes? For most it seemed to be a holiday. Not in the sense of a funfair at Clacton but in the sense of a holy day, time set apart from ordinary life. One sick pilgrim, writing in the newsletter produced by the pilgrimage organisation after her pilgrimage, explained it in precisely those terms: 'this was not merely a pilgrimage, it was a holiday in the original sense of the word, that is a holy day or succession of holy days. I am not a religious person. Nor is Sheila (her companion on the journey), but we both felt exalted by our experience and the wonderful kindness of everyone we met...[1]' What impressed was not, however, the holiness of the pilgrims - none went for solely religious motives such as penance - nor any idea of pious wishes to help 'the less fortunate'. Rather what came over was a desire to go because they expected to enjoy it, to get something out of it. This selfishness of motive was not matched, I must point out immediately, by any selfishness of action on arrival at Lourdes. A few examples, as people speak for themselves may help to give the correct

44

impression. An old lady of eighty said that she went 'to get
away from my telephone and my family - and recharge my
batteries. Spiritually too it's such a refreshment. It's
difficult to tabulate'; a middle aged farmer, one-time
lawyer and one-time trainee priest said, 'It's a real effort
to come. When I come back I say "I'm glad I've been..." I've
been able to help people. I come back renewed in a spiritual
way - (it's) time off to think and pray. Lourdes is very
much a place of kindness and charity'; another old, and
indomitable lady, a former matron at a public school said,
'I go for the good of my soul, a good thing to do, knocks
the selfishness out of you.' A young merchant banker replied
'It's difficult to answer, partly people, partly faith - the
aura of the place, working with the sick, get away from
London. I've got lots of friends going who said it was going
to be fun. You get to know people far more than in London.'

Many of the pilgrims were coming for the second, third,
fourth or even fifth time. The pilgrimage as a whole was
rather unusual. It was organised in connection with
Ampleforth College, a major Catholic public boarding school.
Hence nearly all participants had a connection, however
tenuous, with Ampleforth College and were therefore often
school friends or had a common school lore to draw upon. In
addition, however, there was an astonishing kin network:
forty one percent of the total pilgrims (who numbered 170 in
total in the Ampleforth pilgrimage) had at least one other
kin member on the pilgrimage and if 'the sick' are excluded
from the calculations the number rises to forty nine per
cent (n=132) or nearly half. One can see from this simple
fact why the atmosphere of the pilgrimage was so lively and
animated. For the helpers and for some of the sick the
pilgrimage was a combination of an old boy's reunion and
(extended) family reunion.

The place we were all going to is a small town in the
foothills of the Pyrenees in southern France. In that town
is an internationally renowned Catholic shrine[2]. Its
importance for healing is centred around a grotto, a small
rock cave in which a poor young French girl living near
Lourdes, Bernadette Soubirous, saw eighteen apparitions of a
lady dressed in white between 11 February and 16 July 1858.
The lady spoke eleven times and her messages were usually
simple instructions to Bernadette, e.g. 'Go kiss the ground
as penance for sinners.' In the light of later events three
messages stand out. One was the last message when the lady
said 'I am the immaculate conception,' i.e. that Mary was
conceived free of sin, a dogma that Pius IX had only
declared three years earlier. The other two were that the
lady wanted people to 'come here in procession' and
Bernadette was to 'Go drink at that spring and wash yourself
in it.' There was in fact no spring until Bernadette dug at
the back of the grotto and one burst forth. This spring
provides 32,000 gallons of water a day which is used both
for drinking and for bathing for over three million people
who go hoping to be healed, for, shortly after the spring
appeared, a local man who bathed in it was cured. He was the

first of many. Bernadette herself entered a nunnery and died a nun. She was later canonized.

Today the shrine is administered by the Hospitalite. The Hospitalite is an organisation started in 1880. By tradition it started when a local gentleman saw a cripple trying to reach the shrine and, with a friend, helped him to get there (see Rebsomen, 1930). It became a permanent committee in 1882 with offices sited on a square in the centre of the shrine area. It organises all the events of the shrine by co-ordinating them. Each pilgrimage group has to send a representative to the Hospitalite who acts as a liaison with the group. The work is entirely voluntary and unpaid. In addition to ensuring that there is no conflict over the use of the buildings of the Domaine - the ritual centre of a Lourdes pilgrimage - and the hospices where the sick live, members of the Hospitalite are stationed at the airport and the station to help pilgrims. An individual progresses up the internal hierarchy of the Hospitalite by frequent attendance at the shrine and five visits entitle him to wear leather straps rather than canvas ones. Work for the central Hospitalite is for men and is organised along military lines. Each helper, called a <u>brancadier</u>, wears straps and numbers, given on small buckles on the straps, indicate his grade in the structure. The main function of the Hospitalite is to help the sick pilgrims and this they do by co-ordination and crowd control.

The other important organisation in the shrine is the Bureau Medicale. Set up in 1884, it is also sited on the 'square' and is an organisation of doctors set up to 'test' the claims of cure made at the shrine. They pronounce on the extraordinary nature of cures and require

(1) exact medical diagnosis, i.e. objective medical signs of the disease, not just symptoms, and clear medical signs of its disappearance.
(2) Abnormality in the cure, i.e. the disease should be incurable or the cure needed means which were not used and the cure was rapid with little or no convalescence.

The decision on the miraculous nature of the cure is left to the Church authorities. The Bureau Medicale have extensive medical records on cures, not all of which were declared miraculous, which, following normal medical practice on confidentiality, they release only to qualified doctors. At the time of my visit sixty three cures were recognised as miraculous by the Church (see table below) covering all sorts of diseases including blindness, paralysis, cancer, tuberculosis and multiple sclerosis.

CURES OF LOURDES RECOGNISED AS MIRACULOUS BY THE CHURCH [3]

(List of cures in chronological order)

List N° Actual - Old	NAME and DOMICILE	NATURE of ILLNESS	AGE AT THE DATE OF CURE	DIOCESE AND DATE OF RECOGNITION
1 — 3	Mrs. LATAPIE-CHOUAT Catherine of LOUBAJAC.	Paralysis of cubital type due to traumatic elongation of the brachial plexus for 18 months.	39 years old on 1-3-1858.	
2 — 1	Mr BOURIETTE Louis of LOURDES.	20 years old injury to the right eye with blindness. for 2 years	54 years old in march 1858.	Mandate of Monseigneur Laurence on 18-1-1862.
3 — 2	Mrs. CAZENAVE Blaisette (nee SOUPENE) of LOURDES.	Chemosis or chronic ophthalmitis with ectropion for 3 years.	About 50 years old in march 1858.	
4 — 5	Mr. BUSQUET Henri of NAY.	Adenitis of the root of the neck (undoubtedly tuberculous) with fistulae for 15 months.	About 15 years old on 29-4-1858.	
5 — 4	Mr. BOUHORT Justin of LOURDES.	Chronic post-infective hypothrepsia with retarded motor development. Diagnosis at the time : « consumption. »	2 years old on 6-7-1858.	
6 — 6	Mrs. RIZAN Madeleine of NAY.	Left hemiplegia for 24 years.	About 58 years old on 9-11-1858.	
7 — 7	Miss MOREAU Marie of TARTAS.	Very marked impairment of vision with inflammatory lesions especially of the right eye, progressive for 10 months.	17 years old on 9-11-1858.	
8 — 24	Mr. DE RUDDER Pierre of JABBEKE (Belgium).	Ununited fracture of the leg.	52 years old on 7-4-1875.	Bruges (Belg.) 25-7-1908.
9 — 14	Miss DEHANT Joachime of GEVES (Belgium).	Leg ulcer with extensive gangrene.	29 years old on 13-9-1878.	Namur (Belg.) 25-4-1908.
10 — 37	Miss SEISSON Elisa of ROGNOGNAS.	Hypertrophy of the heart and œdema of the lower limbs.	28 years old on 29-8-1882.	Aix-en-Provence 2-7-1912.
11 — 27	Sister EUGENIA (Marie Mabille) of BERNAY.	Abscess of the true pelvis with vesical and colic fistulae. Bilateral phlebitis.	28 years old on 21-8-1883.	Evreux 30-8-1908.
12 — 36	Sister JULIENNE (Aline Bruyere) of LA ROQUE.	Cavitating pulmonary tuberculosis.	25 years old on 1-9-1889.	Tulle 24-3-1912.
13 — 28	Sister JOSEPHINE-MARIE (Anne JOURDAIN) of GOINCOURT.	Pulmonary tuberculosis.	36 years old on 21-8-1890.	Beauvais 10-10-1908.
14 — 33	Miss CHAGNON Amélie of POITIERS.	Tuberculous osteo-arthritis of the knee and second metatarsal of the foot.	17 years old on 21-8-1891.	Tournai (Belg.) 8-9-1910.
15 — 17	Miss TROUVE Clémentine (Sr Agnès-Marie) of ROUILLE.	Osteo periostitis of the right foot with fistulae.	14 years old on 21-8-1891.	Paris 6-6-1908.
16 — 18	Miss LEBRANCHU Marie of PARIS.	Pulmonary tuberculosis (Koch's bacillae present in sputum).	35 years old on 20-8-1892.	Paris 6-6-1908.
17 — 19	Miss LEMARCHAND Marie of CAEN.	Pulmonary tuberculosis with ulcers of face and leg.	18 years old on 21-8-1892.	Paris 6-6-1908.

List N° Actual - Old	NAME and DOMICILE	NATURE of ILLNESS	AGE AT THE DATE OF CURE	DIOCESE AND DATE OF RECOGNITION
18 / 9	Miss LESAGE Elise of BUCQUOY.	Tuberculous osteo-arthritis of knee.	18 years old on 21-8-1892.	Arras 4-2-1908.
19 / 25	Sister MARIE de la PRESENTATION of LILLE.	Chronic tuberculous gastro-enteritis.	46 years old on 29-8-1892.	Cambrai 15-8-1908.
20 / 12	Father CIRETTE of BEAUMONTEL.	Antero-lateral spinal sclerosis.	46 years old on 31-8-1893.	Evreux 11-2-1908.
21 / 15	Miss HUPRELLE Aurélie of ST-MARTIN-LE-NŒUD.	Apical pulmonary tuberculosis.	26 years old on 21-8-1895.	Beauvais 1-5-1908.
22 / 20	Miss BRACHMANN Esther of PARIS.	Tuberculous peritonitis.	15 years old on 21-8-1896.	Paris 6-6-1908.
23 / 8	Miss TULASNE Jeanne of TOURS.	Lumbar Pott's disease, with neuropathic club foot.	20 years old on 8-9-1897.	Tours 27-10-1907.
24 / 29	Miss MALOT Clémentine of GAUDECHART.	Pulmonary tuberculosis with haemoptysis.	25 years old on 21-8-1898.	Beauvais 1-11-1908.
25 / 21	Mrs. FRANCOIS Rose (nee LABREUVOIES) of PARIS.	Fistular lymphangitis of the right arm with enormous œdema.	36 years old on 20-8-1899.	Paris 6-6-1908.
26 / 22	Reverend Father SALVATOR of DINARD.	Tuberculous peritonitis.	38 years old on 25-6-1900.	Rennes 1-7-1908.
27 / 10	Sister MAXIMILIEN of MARSEILLE.	Hydatid cyst of the liver, phlebitis of the left lower limb.	43 years old on 20-5-1901.	Marseille 5-2-1908.
28 / 26	Miss SAVOYE Marie of CATEAU-CAMBRESIS.	Rheumatic disease of the mitral valve with failure.	24 years old on 20-9-1901.	Cambrai 15-8-1908.
29 / 23	Mrs. BEZENAC Johanna (nee DUBOS) of ST-LAURENT-DES-BATONS.	Pyrexia of unknown origin, impetigo of the eyelids and forehead.	28 years old on 8-8-1904.	Perigueux 2-7-1908.
30 / 16	Sister SAINT-HILAIRE of PEYRELEAU.	Abdominal tumour.	39 years old on 20-8-1904.	Rodez 10-5-1908.
31 / 13	Sister SAINTE-BEATRIX (Rosalie Vildier) of EVREUX.	Laryngo-bronchitis, probably tuberculous.	42 years old on 31-8-1904.	Evreux 25-3-1908.
32 / 11	Miss NOBLET Marie-Thérèse of AVENAY.	Dorso-lumbar spondylitis.	16 years old on 31-8-1905.	Reims 11-2-1908
33 / 34	Miss DOUVILLE DE FRANSSU Cécile of TOURNAI (Belgium).	Tuberculous peritonitis.	19 years old on 21-9-1905.	Versailles 8-12-1909.
34 / 34	Miss MOULIN Antonia of VIENNE.	Osteitic fistulae of the right femur with arthritis of the knee.	30 years old on 10-8-1907.	Grenoble 6-11-1910.
35 / 35	Miss BOREL Marie of MENDE.	Four pyelo-colic fistulae of the lumbar region.	27 years old on 21/22-08-1907	Mende 4-6-1911.
36 / 39	Miss HAUDEBOURG Virginie of LONS-LE-SAULNIER.	Tuberculous cystitis, nephritis.	22 years old on 17-5-1908	Saint-Claude 25-11-1912.
37 / 31	Mrs. BIRE Marie (nee LUCAS) of STE-GEMME-LA-PLAINE.	Blindness of cerebral origin, bilateral optic atrophy.	41 years old on 5-8-1908.	Lucon 30-7-1910.

No.	Name	Disease	Cured	Place and date
38	Miss ALLOPE Aimée of VERN.	Numerous tuberculous abscesses with 4 fistulae of the anterior abdominal parietis.	37 years old on 28-5-1909.	Angers 5-8-1910.
39	Miss ORION Juliette of ST-HILAIRE-DE-VOUST.	Pulmonary and laryngeal tuberculosis, suppurating left mastoiditis.	24 years old on 22-7-1910.	Luçon 18-10-1913.
40	Mrs. FABRE Marie of MONTREDON.	Muco-membranous enteritis, uterine prolapse.	32 years old on 26-9-1911	Cahors 8-9-1912.
41	Miss BRESSOLES Henriette of NICE.	Pott's disease, paraplegia.	28 years old on 3-7-1924.	Nice 4-6-1957.
42	Miss BROSSE Lydia of ST-RAPHAEL.	Multiple tuberculous fistulae with wide undermining.	41 years old on 11-10-1930.	Coutances 5-8-1958.
43	Sister MARIE-MARGUERITE (Françoise Capitaine) of RENNES.	Abscess of the left kidney with phlyctenular œdema and «cardiac crises.»	64 years old on 22-1-1937.	Rennes 20-5-1946.
44	Miss JAMAIN Louise of PARIS.	Pulmonary, intestinal and peritoneal tuberculosis.	22 years old on 1-4-1937.	Paris 14-12-1951.
45	Mr. PASCAL Francis of BEAUCAIRE.	Blindness, paralysis of the lower limbs.	3 years 10 months on 28-8-1938.	Aix-en-Provence 31-5-1949.
46	Miss CLAUZEL Gabrielle of ORAN.	Rheumatic spondylitis.	49 years old on 15-8-1943.	Oran 18-3-1948.
47	Miss FOURNIER Yvonne of LIMOGES.	Extending and progressive post-traumatic syndrome (Leriche's syndrome).	22 years old on 19-8-1945.	Paris 14-11-1959.
48	Mrs. MARTIN Rose of NICE.	Cancer of the uterine cervix (epithelioma of the cylindrical glands).	45 years old on 3-7-1947.	Nice 5-5-1949.
49	Mrs. GESTAS Jeanne (nee PELIN) of BEGLES.	Dyspeptic troubles with obstructive episodes.	50 years old on 22-8-1947.	Bordeaux 13-7-1952.
50	Miss CANIN Marie-Thérèse of MARSEILLE.	Dorso-lumbar Pott's disease and tuberculous peritonitis with fistulae.	37 years old on 9-10-1947.	Marseille 6-6-1952.
51	Miss CARINI Maddelena of SAN REMO.	Peritoneal, pleuro-pulmonary and bony tuberculosis with coronary disease.	31 years old on 15-8-1948.	Milan (Italy) 2-6-1960.
52	Miss FRETEL Jeanne of RENNES.	Tuberculous peritonitis.	34 years old on 8-10-1948.	Rennes 20-11-1950.
53	Miss THEA Angele (Sr Marie-Mercedes) of TETTNAG (Germany).	Multiple sclerosis for six years.	29 years old on 20-5-1950.	Tarbes-Lourdes 28-6-1961.
54	Mr. GANORA Evasio of CASALE (Italy).	Hodgkin's disease.	37 years old on 2-6-1950.	Casale (Italy) 31-5-1955.
55	Miss FULDA Edeltraut of WIEN (Austria).	Addison's disease.	34 years old on 12-8-1950.	Wien (Austria) 18-5-1955.
56	Mr. PELLEGRIN Paul of TOULON.	Post-operative fistula following a liver abscess.	52 years old on 3-10-1950.	Frejus-Toulon 8-12-1953.
57	Brother SCHWAGER Léo of FRIBOURG (Switzerland).	Multiple sclerosis for 5 years.	28 years old on 30-4-1952.	Lausanne-G.-F. 18-12-1960.
58	Mrs. COUTEAULT Alice (nee GOURDON) of BOUILLE-LORETZ.	Multiple sclerosis for 3 years.	35 years old on 16-5-1952.	Poitiers 16-7-1956.
59	Miss BIGOT Marie of LA RICHARDAIS.	Arachnoiditis of the posterior fossa (blindness, deafness, hemiplegia).	31 years old on 10-10-1954.	Rennes 15-8-1956.

List N° Actual - Old	NAME and DOMICILE	NATURE of ILLNESS	AGE AT THE DATE OF CURE	DIOCESE AND DATE OF RECOGNITION
60	60	Miss NOUVEL Ginette of CARMAUX.	Budd-Chiari disease (supra-hepatic venous thrombosis).	26 years old on 23-9-1954.	Albi 23-1-1963.
61	62	Miss ALOI Elisa of PATTI (Italy).	Tuberculous osteo-arthritis with fistulae at numerous sites on the right lower limb.	27 years old on 5-6-1958.	Messine (Italy) 26-5-1965.
62	61	Miss TAMBURINI Juliette of MARSEILLE.	Femoral osteoperiostitis with fistulae, epistaxis, for ten years.	23 years old on 17-7-1959.	Marseille 11-5-1965.
63	—	Mr. MICHELI Vittorio of SCURELLE (Italy).	Sarcoma of Pelvis.	23 years old on 1-6-1963.	Trento 26-5-1976.

The Bureau Medicale as well as distributing the list of miraculous cures given above also distribute, on request, individual case studies. A typical example (case 54 on the above table) was the account they gave of the miraculous healing of Mr Ganora (a pseudonym). He was diagnosed as suffering from Hodgkin's disease in February 1950 after exhaustive diagnostic tests taken during the previous month and he expected to die. However he came to Lourdes on 31 May of that year and upon immersion in the water felt a great warmth course through his body. He rose from the baths and walked back to the hospital where he acted as a stretcher-bearer during the rest of his stay in Lourdes. When he was examined at the Bureau Medicale his fever had gone and his liver, spleen and glands were no longer palpable - there were no signs of the disease. He went home from Lourdes and returned to his old occupation of a farm labourer. In 1953 his own doctor testified to his continued good health and in 1954 he was given another full examination by the Bureau Medicale who could find no abnormalities. He was finally examined by an International Medical Committee in Paris, who confirmed his good health in 1955. The original histological specimens, taken in 1950 were re-examined and the initial diagnosis of Hodgkin's disease was confirmed. Having survived in good health almost five years from the date of his initial examination by the Bureau Medicale he was, so far as the medical profession was concerned, cured (five years being the standard criteria of cure amongst doctors) and on 31 May 1955, five years to the day since he stepped into the baths at Lourdes an ecclesiastical court pronounced his cure as miraculous.

I arrived at Lourdes on a Friday but I want to start my account on the following Sunday (to cover the full week would require an inordinate amount of description) because the Sunday, Monday and Tuesday were the central three days of a seven day pilgrimage and all the essential observations which help in understanding the pilgrimage were made on these three days.

By Sunday I had settled into the routine of the pilgrimage and been allocated to a team of helpers. As was intimated above, in the comments on the kin relationships, there was a fundamental division between 'the sick' and the helpers. 'The sick' were housed in a building resembling a hospital in many respects, with wards of various sizes but with no operating theatre or similar facilities. In fact when one of our sick was taken seriously ill she had to be moved to hospital. There were two doctors and two nurses for our sick, all of whom were members of the pilgrimage. The hospital was run by nuns who provided the building, food and linen. The wards were divided into male and female, separate from each other but nearby. The windows in the ward were high up but standing one could look out over the town of Lourdes with a particularly good view of the castle. The helpers were housed in nearby hotels. Just as the sick were divided into male and female so were the helpers. The 'Lady Helpers' - the title they were given - did the cooking and the washing of the sick. The male helpers or brancadiers - the title we were given - did the lifting of the sick, the towing of the invalid chairs and the general fetching and carrying. This division was not however rigidly adhered to, some of the hefty girls being much better at lifting than me! The helpers worked in teams of six, with a leader, for a shift period. The shifts were posted daily by the team leader. The brancadiers wear straps of canvas, which look somewhat like the braces of lederhosen and form part of a well organised system whereby they take orders from a 'leather-belt', a brancadier who has qualified by being at Lourdes for five weeks, working for the central organisation of the Hospitalite to be a leader. Brancadiers engage in crowd control on the 'Domaine' - control that is very necessary when there are up to 30,000 people in a small area.

The principal buildings and areas of the Domaine are on and by a main square in front of a large basilica church. The square is enclosed on two sides by ramps which lead up to the upper stories of the church. Beyond the square is the river Gave. Along the Gave there is an embankment from which one can view the grotto which is the central religious point within the Domaine. The grotto is merely a small cleft in the rocks of a river cliff. At the top of the cliff rears the side of the basilica. Beyond the grotto are the baths, an unpretentious block of buildings. Across the Gave is a field, known as the 'Prairie' from which, once a bridge is crossed, one can look back at the grotto and the baths. From the grotto to the edge of the Domaine there is a tarmacadamed processional route which comes back towards the square alongside a huge grass covered mound which is the underground basilica. In the Domaine in addition to the buildings already mentioned, stand a hospice, a modern chapel dedicated to St Joseph and administrative buildings of which the most prominent is that of the Bureau Medicale.

So the sick, the lady helpers and the brancadiers form the main characters, as it were, in this story. Sunday morning, one brancadier, me, got out of bed at 6.45 a.m. - I was lucky our team was on the late shift that day, another team had been in the wards since 5.30 a.m. - went downstairs and had breakfast in the hotel and then grabbed my straps and made my way the short distance to the hospital and climbed to the third floor past the Belgian miners' ward where all the male helpers wear blue boiler suits and miners' helmets. (On my first day there they'd been operating the lifts and seeing them wearing hard hats, not knowing about the Belgian miners, I'd half thought the lifts were rather dangerous!) Then into the ward. Breakfast was being cleared up and I joined in as the first shift knocked off for breakfast, clearing plates, chatting to the sick, helping them to the toilet, helping them dress, and about eight o'clock, starting to get them into little blue metal chairs which had wheels on the back. You jammed your foot on the front, got your arms round the sick person with their arms around you, and hoisted them into the chair. It's a knack, but even when you've got it, killing on the back muscles. Then the chairs were tipped back and the sick wheeled to the lift, into the lift, and out at ground floor level into blue 'voitures'. The nearest description I can give of them is that they closely resemble a rickshaw with the brancadier providing the coolie power. When all were ready we set off along a specially marked route through the town and into the Domaine. There, when we had gone down the spiral ramp to the centre of the underground basilica the voitures were taken from us by leatherbelts and arranged in rows. When this vast underground cavern, resembling an upturned boat or the inside of a whale, the size of a medieval cathedral was full to bursting - the only ones sitting down were some people on a few benches, the sick in their voitures, the choir and church dignitaries - high mass began. I won't try to describe it in detail - only to stress that it was a beautiful ritual performance combining swirls of colour as the priests in their different robes entered the basilica in procession and flowed (and I use the word 'flowed' deliberately) around the altar. The movement of priests around the altar during the mass was like watching a slow motion film of a flower unfolding its petals. The mass took place to the accompaniment of singing from an excellent choir before thousands of people surrounding the central altar.

After high mass the sick were returned to the wards (with all the loading and unloading involved), then loaded back again to go to St Joseph's chapel for a short service of absolution conducted entirely by and for the pilgrimage. From there they viewed the Blessed Sacrament Procession (or as the young helpers called it - BSP). All the pilgrims had taken part in it the day before.

This starts from the grotto. Each contingent carries a banner identifying itself. Then, to the accompaniment of hymns and prayers in different languages led by tannoyed voices, the procession finally gets under way. It goes from the grotto, along a special processional route which takes it away from the basilica until it reaches the limits of the Domaine. It then turns around and proceeds back toward the central square in front of the basilica. The tail has only just started when the front is finishing. When they get to the square the central banner (of the last supper), brought by the Belgian miners at this pilgrimage week, is held on top of the steps and the other banners go up the steps to either side giving a very medieval effect. Whenever the sacrament passes during the procession people kneel. There is no difficulty in knowing where it is because it is held by a bishop and he, and the sacrament, are shielded by a canopy supported on four poles. When the host arrives in the square it is taken up onto the steps and the doctors of the Bureau Medicale who have taken part in the procession kneel on the steps. The priest says 'Lord he whom you love is sick. Lord say the word and I shall be healed' in several languages. This is repeated by the congregation. The Kyrie is sung and the host is taken around the square and displayed to the sick. Then the host is taken into the church to the singing of alleluia.

As the host disappears the carefully buit-up structure of the ritual collapses and the people crush and mix to get out of the Domaine. The sick are not taken back in procession, but make their own way back with a <u>brancadier</u> towing them, stopping to shop for souveniers - Lourdes water bottles, crucifixes, etc. - and/or have a drink in the pavement cafes (<u>brancadiers</u> are, incidentally, required to remove their straps when sitting in a cafe).

After supper the unloading and loading sequence takes place again as the sick are taken to the torch light procession. This follows the same route as the BSP but torches are carried and the repetitive Ave Maria is sung. The sick are taken back and put to bed and the helpers go off and drink and talk until the early hours of the morning.

Monday was a very long day for me because I was on night duty, but I want to concentrate on the rest of the day because that was when I was a helper at the baths and no account of Lourdes is complete without an account of the baths. As a writer in the pilgrimage newsletter expressed it 'the bath has become so central in the phenomenon of Lourdes that no visit is really complete without one'[4]. On arrival at the baths I was registered with the Hospitalite and then went upstairs, put on a large blue apron, took off my socks and rolled up my trousers and then went downstairs again with the others, most of whom were Italian and I believe (one of our group could speak Italian) medical students.

The baths were laid out as a row of cubicles, each about the size of a small room with a shower curtain at one end, chairs and hooks at either side, separated from the next cubicle by the curtains. At the far end of each room was a stone bath with steps and rails on either side of it. All of us stood inside a cubicle and the <u>chef</u> of the baths said a short prayer. After the prayer most of the helpers wanted to work in the cubicles that dealt with the sick who needed assistance. (There are six cubicles, I think, one for the walking sick, one for children - which is separated by a glass door - and the remaining four for the invalids.) As people came in they either undressed themselves or were helped to undress by the attendants. There are six or so attendants per cubicle, usually arranged to give a spread of languages. In the morning I was in a cubicle for the walking sick but in the afternoon I managed to get into one for invalids, so I could see the difference, only to find myself the only French speaker among Italians, and my French is atrocious! The sick person is undressed to their underpants (I'm talking of men, of course) leaving their clothes on a chair or a hook. They then go behind a curtain at the side of the bath and a blue linen towel, continuously wet after the first person has used it, is wrapped around them and they take off their underpants. They are helped or carried - there are special crude contrivances for taking people who

can only sit or lie - down the steps into the water to the
far end of the bath. The water is very cold. It comes from
the underground spring in the grotto revealed by St
Bernadette. Interestingly 'in the apparitions to Bernadette
Our Lady did not tell anyone to bathe in the waters; she
told them to drink'[4]. They then cross themselves and say
in their own language 'St Bernadette pray for us, Mary pray
for us.' Then two men, one on either side, hold them and
lower them backward into the water with their arms crossed
on their chest. If the sick person asks for it they're given
complete immersion and also offered a cup of the water from
the bath to drink. They then kiss a statuette of 'Our Lady'
and are helped back up the steps, get their towels off and
underpants on, are dressed - or dress themselves - without
drying and go out. People queue for hours for this
immersion.

I should mention that the water is not changed during the
day and although the sick are bathing with all sorts of open
wounds and infectious diseases, none have been known to
catch the diseases of others. At the end of the day the bath
attendants can have a dip themselves as a special privilege
- one that I took. I wasn't going to drink the water
however but when I opened my mouth to tell the boys holding
me they put me under, so I drank it willy-nilly!

Because of my night duty I spent the morning of the
Tuesday in bed but got up in time to join the trek to the
Cite de Secours. This is a collection of buildings outside
Lourdes for those who are too poor to stay in Lourdes yet
still wish to come on a pilgrimage. On previous days we had
all dressed formally - even in the heat of Southern France -
because we had been taking the sick to the Domaine which was
sacred ground, in the sense that a church is sacred ground,
so we had to wear socks, ties and jackets. On that Tuesday
however were all dressed informally, not to say
ridiculously, in shorts, sun hats, Hawaiian beach shirts and
the like. We towed the voitures (two helpers to each) up a
very steep hill - stopping halfway for drinks and ice-creams
- and we needed them. The hill was one in four in short
sections and that's quite a slope to pull up a rickshaw. On
arrival at the Cite de Secours we sat around under some
trees in a natural amphitheatre (it was created
'naturalness', much on the lines of Japanese gardens) hiding
from the sun. Facing us was an altar. A mass was then held
and after the mass each sick person was anointed with oil
while helpers placed their hands upon them. This was the key
ritual of the week for the Ampleforth pilgrimage and in his
sermon at the amphitheatre one of the priests said this. I
will give you a synopsis of his sermon because sermons are
something I've missed out so far and this sermon was
considered to be an important one by the helpers and the
sick. He said:

> Lourdes exists, Christ lives, to change people, to
> heal people, not only physically but also
> spiritually. We have had absolution (this was a
> reference to the service in St Joseph's chapel),

everything has been forgiven, everything forgotten-
...we have been made whole...the service of anointing
is a renewal of our baptismal vows, a conversion from
an old way of life to a new way of life. The central
act of the pilgrimage is the anointing of the sick.
The power of Christ is still present because Christ
is present. The days of miracles have not ended. We
are like the men who carried the young man with
determination to Christ. They took the roof off. We
too have been determined and carried our sick up the
hill to Christ. He renewed the spirit of the
paralysed man. He will renew your spirit...Lourdes is
the curing of the spirit first of all. That is
immeasurably more important than the curing of the
body. After our Lord cured the spirit he then cured
the body. The power of Christ will come to you if
that is his will. But you must believe in the power
of Christ...there must be total acceptance of his
will.

I didn't see any miracles during my visit. What I did see
however were marginal changes in some people's functioning,
e.g. one man who had at the beginning of the week travelled
in a _voiture_ was by the end of the week pulling his own
empty _voiture_. The best example of an improvement in
functioning was perhaps Joan[5]. She was a paraplegic and it
is useful in this respect to compare her with Marie who was
also a paraplegic. Joan was a northern working-class woman
who was not a Catholic. She had come on the pilgrimage
because the Catholic priest who had visited when she was in
hospital and had kept up his visits afterwards had finally
arranged for her to come to Lourdes. She was withdrawn and
uncommunicative on arrival. This was hardly surprising,
since at home she spent most of her days sitting watching
television by herself in a house that was empty during the
day because all the family worked. In addition the helpers
on the pilgrimage were upper class and must have appeared as
strangers to her. She had some movement of her arms but
could not feed herself or give herself drinks. Marie was
better off in this respect having full movement of her arms.
In England she was a resident of a Cheshire home, married to
a fellow resident, and acted as the representative of the
sick people in the home on the house committee. She had no
difficulty in communicating with the helpers, and being a
Canadian was not seen in class terms.

By the end of the week there was no improvement in Marie,
who in spite of her Catholicism had not enjoyed Lourdes and
vowed never to come again. Joan on the other hand was able
to lift her drinks to her mouth, particularly her 'glass of
stout', and was seriously considering becoming a Catholic.
She was also a joy to be with and spent her time laughing
and joking with the helpers. Marie has been contrasted with
Joan to demonstrate that although some showed improvement in
functioning it was not true of all and nor was it
necessarily those you would most expect to improve who did
so.

'The power of Christ will come to you if that is his will. But you must believe in the power of Christ...there must be total acceptance of his will' said the priest in his sermon at the Cite de Secours and encapsulated in two sentences the Christian ideal of healing. The rest of this chapter can be viewed as a commentary upon these sentences, an attempt to spell out in detail the implications of them. This commentary includes examples drawn from other Christian healing centres and brings witchcraft back into consideration. The key words in the sentences are 'power' and 'will'. Healing for the Christian comes from the intervention of a will-full power (in this context, I mean a power literally 'full of will') and for that power to operate the sick person must give up his or her own will to the power of God. It is however not enough to demonstrate a belief in a will-full power and a will-less person as integral parts of Christian healing. What must be examined also is the way the gap between the will-full power and the will-less person is bridged. How is the power brought to bear upon the sick person? What are the channels of God's grace, to use the language of the believers? These channels are people and places, people as individual healers or as the community of believers, and places as shrines. But it is not sufficient to bring a group of people together or to stand in a shrine to become a channel for the power of God. There must also be prayer and rituals to open the channels to God's power. Precisely how this is achieved at Lourdes we will return to later, but first, to more fully understand the notions of 'power' and 'will', it is necessary to look at some other Christian healers.

BURRSWOOD

There's a very good pub at Groombridge – typical English Tourist Board style – on the village green across from the church and serving good food as well as good beer. Burrswood is located in that sort of area – 'rural' England where there are farms but whose fields seem to be full of ponies for the daughters of the local commuters. Burrswood itself is sited just ouside the hamlet, down a track. It's a large country house built in stone in the late Elizabethan style. At the side of the house there is a church which outside resembles a parish church of the Early English period but inside, with its religious statues, paintings and painted ceiling, is much more like a catholic church in Italy. The inside of the house is in keeping with its external appearance and has wood-panelled walls and polished floors. In fact, like the pub in the village, it could easily pass muster by the British Tourist Board as a traditional English hotel, but for the religious objects which are evident in every room.

Any account of Burrswood must briefly review Dorothy Kerin's life as it is in large measure a product of her energy and vision. The photographs of her (in the publicity material distributed by Burrswood) show her as a short middle-aged lady with a flowered print dress, pearl necklace and a perm covered by a hat or the headdress she often wore. Her expression is somewhat dreamy and her smile is enigmatic.

She recovered from tuberculosis in a miraculous manner in February 1912 when during one night she reached a crisis and the next day was cured, a cure confirmed by x-rays. In June she went to London and made a statement to a newspaper. It included the following statements:

> In my restoration to health I have been entrusted with a message to the whole world, a promise of healing to the sick, comfort to the sorrowing and faith to the faithless... How these things are going to be brought into practice has not been revealed to me yet...
> I know that it was not for me alone but that there is a Divine purpose in my being singled out to manifest the healing power of the Spirit...I am an instrument in God's hands. I know that He closed my human eyes and ears so that I might receive his message. He took my conscious self away for a time, so that I might know spiritual things[6].

This pattern of illness and cure was repeated three or four times in her life. In 1930 she founded Chapel House, Ealing, as a nursing home which ultimately grew and moved to become Burrswood, at that time derelict. The house was renovated and in 1959, in response to a vision, a church was built at the side of the house:

> I saw in the rose garden here a Church. There it stood in all its strength and beauty. Out of the windows there streamed a golden light, lighting up eveything it touched. As I watched I noticed that this light came from within. Then I heard the Voice, that I had learned to know, saying, 'Build this Church for me'[6].

The first plan drawn up did not correspond to her vision so it was modified and the church built, in eleven months, by a small firm of local builders and was completed in 1960. She died in January 1963 after choosing Dr Aubert as her successor.

Today[7] Burrswood is a charitable trust which runs a nursing home. The fees charged are low and one in four come for nothing. There are 36 beds and the average stay is about a fortnight which gives a turnover of about 1,000 people a year. There are three healing services a week, all open to the public. There's no emotionalism at these services, they're quiet Anglican services. (A description of a typical Anglican healing service is given in the account of the Ecumenical Centre p.60.)

Patients are largely middle-class women but a bursary means that others can come. In addition there is a special bursary fund from the Rank Organisation which enables them to accommodate leukaemic children and their parents.

The staff consist of the warden and physician (Ken Cuming), secretarial staff and nursing staff (who are paid below normal rates to keep costs down). The selection of patients is done by a booking committee consisting of the warden, two senior nurses and the bookings secretary (who is an ex-nursing sister). Every letter of application is considered. To ensure the nurses are not overburdened those needing heavy nursing are kept small in number and psychiatric cases are refused (they have no psychiatric nurses and the home is not licensed for acute psychiatric cases).

A patient normally receives breakfast in bed in their own private room. Then they are bathed and dressed, after which the doctor visits them if needed. If they are mobile they are encouraged to get up and go outdoors (the house has beautiful and extensive grounds). There is morning coffee and lunch outdoors if it is a good day. On Sundays there is tea from a silver tea-service. During the day the patients are taken for walks, have their posture corrected and receive massage as necessary.

The warden's day starts with a communion service. There is then a conference in his room with the nursing staff, chaplain and the physiotherapist where the night report on each patient is presented. On Mondays and Fridays the domestic staff assemble for prayers and either meditation (Fridays) or readings (Monday). The warden, in his capacity as a doctor, then goes to see the patients. On completion of that he opens the post before going on some visits in the local area. During the afternoon there is a two-hour quiet period followed by an outpatient clinic for those who have made an appointment. The day concludes with tea followed by hostesses visiting the patients. These are women who worked with Dorothy Kerin and they still come in to chat to patients.

AN ECUMENICAL CENTRE[8]

Burrswood, like Lourdes, has facilities for patients to stay a period of time. It is a nursing home. Not all Christian healing is undertaken in this way however. Much more common is the practice of holding healing services in a church open to all who wish to come. This was the practice at a large Victorian church in a decaying area of a market city in England. In fact the area was being rebuilt at the time of my visits to the church and I remember it as one of the few static points in an area where whole streets of terraced homes disappeared into piles of rubble and were replaced by red-brick modern council maisonettes. This process meant that a lot of building materials, building equipment and mud were left lying around the approach roads to the church. At this church:

> Early in 1973 the decision was made to establish a Counselling and Healing Centre in what were near derelict buildings adjoining...The Healing Ministry of the Vicar...was active, the premises available, together with a loan of 6,000 pounds to convert them...
> The idea was to set up an independent organisation of Christian people offering help to all who were in need regardless of their beliefs and without charge; to accept the discipline of the Church of all denominations on a completely ecumenical basis...
> The chapel is in regular daily use for intercessions and for individual anointing and laying-on-of-hands. The Healing Services in (the) Church are an important part of the combined life of the church and centre[9].

The healing services held at the church followed the conventions of the Anglican Church and were held once a month. They consisted of hymn singing, readings from the Bible and a sermon. All these were in some way related to healing. For example, in one sermon the priest talked about Dorothy Kerin and then went on to say

> The world regards death as the ultimate failure and defeat...Death is the ultimate healing. The ministry of healing opens the way to a marvellous and radiant death...The message is that we are all in God's hands. Each one of us is also part of the community. We are the body of Christ. Christ is a healer. We are therefore healers. We are not doing something ourselves we are opening ourselves to the power flowing through us...God is concerned with the whole man not just physical healing - healing in your mind, body and spirit. The touch of Jesus will aid us just as it raised Dorothy Kerin. The same hand is with us. You and I must empty ourselves and make ourselves open to the power and love of the risen healing Christ.

In addition there was a period of intercession when a large list of names[10] was read out by several priests and a lay reader and healing was asked for them. The high point of the service was the laying on of hands by the four attendants. This was conducted as communion is conducted in the Anglican Church, i.e. people queued silently awaiting their turn at the altar-rail behind which the four officiants moved.

Anointing at the healing centre adjoining the church was a much less frequent act of healing except during special children's services held in the chapel of the healing centre. The major activity of the healing centre appeared to be non-directive counselling conducted in rooms set aside for that purpose. However, I did observe one anointing of an adult.

I'd arrived at the centre one morning (I made a habit of popping in whenever I had some spare time) and the warden greeted me with 'You've arrived just in time for an anointing.' He told me that the man, who was elderly, was depressed and had been brought by his brother. He then telephoned for the priest to come over (the vicarage is next door to the centre). While we were waiting for the priest we went into the chapel where the man broke down and wept. The warden said 'good, good'. The priest arrived and chairs were arranged so that the officiants faced the man and his brother. Interestingly the brother and Bill[11] sat with one empty seat between them, a pattern which the officiants mimicked. The warden then told the priest,

> The man is worried, he lives alone and has done for seventeen years. He's a proud man, worried about the fact that when he was confirmed he was more worried about his hair than the ceremony. He keeps getting up in the night to comb his hair. (He was nearly bald.) Also he has a thing about lifts.

he concluded by saying 'People get these phobias.'

The priest then told Bill 'anointing doesn't involve a loss of free will. You must lose your self. He's been -' Bill interjected with 'selfish'. The priest then went on to stress that anointing is nothing unusual. He got a Bible and read the passage 'when a man is ill he must get the elders of the church to anoint him', stressing the word 'must'. Bill said he was an Anglican and the warden told him that we were all Anglicans. The priest then explained the laying on of hands and suggested the brother also did it. He then explained that oil is a symbol of consecration and rehallowing, consecrated by the bishop, and read a letter of thanks from a woman who had been anointed and was able to eat properly, something she hadn't been able to do before. Prayers were said, with all kneeling, stressing opening up to the Holy Spirit and then the priest stood and made the sign of the cross with oil on the forehead of Bill. All remained kneeling while another prayer was said about driving out evil, particularly the evil of pride, and bringing Bill into the care and protection of Jesus; then the warden and the priest laid on hands (the brother did not participate). The warden talked once again about pride and stressed that Bill was being received into Jesus. Finally they all said the Lord's prayer together. As they stood to go out the warden squeezed Bill's arm.

After leaving the chapel we all had tea and Bill gave five pounds to the lift fund. The priest told Bill and his brother that healing is a process and relapses may occur. Bill's brother said he'd just brought Bill, hadn't told him where he was going. Bill asked if they knew anyone in Birmingham who did healing (he lived in Birmingham). They

discussed this and after discovering his old vicar was a
friend of the warden, the warden went off to 'phone him and
came back with the name of a vicar in that area of
Birmingham who held healing services. The brother then told
them that his wife was nervous and they suggested he brought
her along. He said she wouldn't come and they told him not
to tell her where she was going. They also told him about a
woman cured of 'nerves' who was now off valium tablets. He
considered that marvellous.

One of the interesting things I noticed throughout this
ritual of anointing and the events preceding and following
it was that Bill was 'socially distanced'. The others talked
about him as though he were not present; they shook hands
with his brother but not with him and never made eye-contact
with him for any sustained period of time. In short they
treated him like a child.

SUFFERING, WHOLENESS AND WILL

The Christian concept of healing, as I argued earlier, sees
God as a will-full power who intervenes in this world to
produce change in the sick person. God is also seen as
omnipotent. But if God is an omnipotent will-full power why
then is there illness at all? This problem, in religious
terminology the problem of theodicy, is an important aspect
of the thinking of those involved in Christian healing.
Various solutions are open to the Christian. The traditional
solution has been to blame Satan. Interestingly, neither at
Burrswood nor at the Ecumenical healing centre, nor at
Lourdes, was this option taken. One option that was taken
was to blame mankind. The individual sick person could not
be blamed; illness is a type of deviance for which the
individual is not held responsible. Responsibility has
therefore to be assigned elsewhere, to other men. In the
Philippines, as we have seen, that is what accusations of
witchcraft achieve. In England responsibility may be
assigned to ancestors rather than to neighbours:

> I'm sure God never gave diseases to anybody. I'm sure
> it's something we brought upon ourselves. Having said
> that I think it becomes more involved...I think Jesus
> himself did say 'sins unto the third and fourth
> generation' and there may well be people being born
> with muscular dystrophy or multiple sclerosis
> or...mongols and so forth when it probably wasn't the
> fault of the father and mother at all...it may go
> back quite a long time. One has to get this
> perspective which is two-fold. One, that in God's
> eyes, in Christ's eyes, you can commit a sin and
> kneel down, or whatever, and say 'I repent of my sins
> please forgive me' and receive absolution and this
> can all be done in a matter of minutes. That's one
> part of the exercise but the other part of the
> exercise is the law of karma or the law of 'as ye
> sow, so shall ye reap' and I think that's what

applies to the third and fourth generation... That
karma, that the world has brought upon itself has got
to be worked out of the system...and (that's) not
generally something you can do too quickly[12].

An interesting variant of this idea was provided by a
trustee of the Ecumenical healing centre who was also a
medical doctor:

Disease is a manifestation of evilness. I don't mean
individual evilness, although this can happen...you
can cause illness yourself by behaving badly...but I
think that Albert Schweitzer was the first to coin
the phrase 'collective evilness of men'. Over the
millennia man has behaved so badly towards his fellow
creatures.
    Let me explain this by example. It may well have
been that the tubercule bacillus might have, many
thousands of years ago, been a symbiotic organism,
like most other organisms...I could visualize a state
where the tubercule bacillus because of man's
behaviour had no alternative but to take on the role
that it has. Pathological organisms have come about
because of man's collective evilness in the past.

An alternative explanation adds a psychoanalytic twist to
the notion by seeing illness as in part a consequence of the
Jungian collective unconsciousness and in part a consequence
of past modes of life:

The healing ministry has much to do with the healing
of the memory. There are four areas: physical,
mental, emotional and spiritual.
    The body has memories, the lines on faces are the
body's memories, a record of our total experience.
Nothing happens to us that isn't registered on us.
The body registers the memory of experience although
we can't always recall it. It is often expressed in
particular illnesses. What does this illness mean,
what is it saying? It is the body expressing some
kind of experience.
    (Turning to the mental) The way we happened to be
educated is part of what we are.. My thinking is
based on memories. The mind too is an area of memory
on which our experience is registered.
    This is particularly true of the emotional parts of
our life. Some is conscious. What psychologists have
told us is that a lot of what we can feel is
remembered unconsciously. We have forgotten things,
suppressed things, but it is still there. In some
circumstances we feel discomfort because the
unconscious is activated. We also have what Jung
called the collective unconscious. We inherit
something of our whole history of humanity and
cultural background. In Christian doctrine the same
thing is expressed by the fall. There are aspects of
ourselves that we inherit. We have something of the

weight of humanity.
    When we look at the spiritual, guilt is relevant
here - the soul area of our being. The Christian
doctrine of forgiveness is the greatest doctrine of
all.
    (Illness) is in body, mind, emotions, soul - there
are memories to be healed in every one of these
areas.
    (We) accept that an awful lot of illness is
psychosomatic. A lot of illness has its roots in the
soul[13].

The viewpoint presented here is that the individual as he
is now cannot be blamed for his illness, although his past,
perhaps his childhood, may be causing the illness he now
suffers from.

All the explanations for suffering we have looked at so
far have stressed that suffering and affliction come not
from God but man's behaviour. However, there is within the
Christian tradition a view of suffering that sees it not as
a blemish in God's plans but as a part of them. Suffering is
a means of developing people so that they shall be more
Christ-like. Although not a major theme amongst the healers
I studied, this idea was expressed in a sermon at Lourdes
where a priest suggested that 'the sick' were more worthy
than the helpers because of their suffering, and a former
warden of Burrswood expressed a similar idea in his
writings:

    I am not advocating suffering for its own sake, which
    is a morbid idea: what I am saying is that if
    suffering has to be faced, the knowledge that the
    struggle against it is not meaningless, but is an
    opportunity for developing qualities such as courage
    and bravery, can turn a seemingly hopeless situation
    into a challenge...And if it is true that the soul
    survives the death of the body, qualities such as
    courage - which are not physical but spiritual -
    become the soul's permanent acquisitions. But for
    those who believe that physical health is all
    important, and who identify themselves with their
    bodies, illness and death have virtually no redeeming
    features[14].

The concern with the problem of suffering, although
present amongst Christians involved in healing, is not of
major interest to Christian healers. What they are much more
concerned with is trying to understand what healing achieves
and trying to see how the healing power of God may reach
those in need.

For nearly all Christians involved in healing the central
concern is not with physical healing but with healing of the
'whole person'. As we have seen, healing may be considered
to have taken place when death has occurred; relief of
symptoms is not seen as sufficient: 'The healing ministry is

ministry to wholeness. We cannot break man up and treat the parts. The healing ministry must have interrelation of those four parts - physical, mental, emotional and spiritual - always recognised. Symptom relief is not enough[13].'

A point of view echoed by the chaplain at the Ecumenical healing centre:

I see healing as wholeness. I'm reluctant to emphasize just physical healing. We're so interrelated as human beings, and in different parts of ourselves. Any physical healing may be the last link in the chain...wholeness of body, mind and spirit. To be complete one needs the right relationship in three directions. The right relationship with God, the right relationship with other people and indeed the right relationship with oneself.

Some, in fact, see healing merely as part of an evangelical mission - a way of witnessing to God's power. Thus the warden of the Ecumenical healing centre said:

They might come to be healed but that's not how we look at it...They're looking for something, it may be spiritual, and that's the opportunity to put before them the possibility of a sort of wholeness of life, a purpose in life, that helps it to relate...The ultimate aim is always that you can help them realise there is a God...If they were brought closer into harmony with God they would be able to get straight to deal with some of their problems.

And one of the trustees, when asked by me about the results of healing, replied:

People always say, 'What are the results of this?' I don't think anybody knows. I mean, occasionally you have a result and people are much better. The real result is an inner thing...I think this is where so many people get disappointed and they get bogged down with healing because they expect results. I remember a child with a tumour who didn't get well. But there was the most wonderful sort of healing in that house...we were able to almost become a team with God in helping the child. No bitterness involved. Suddenly we all saw it at the same moment, that this was what healing was all about. That she was, in a sense, sent for some reason and the reason was that the parents should begin to understand.

And another trustee, closely involved in the charismatic renewal within the Anglican church, was even more specific:

There are three elements missing from the established, furred-up pipes of the present established Church (quoting from the Bible):

"Faith will bring with it these miracles: believers will cast out devils in my name and speak in strange tongues; if they handle snakes or drink any deadly poison, they will come to no harm; and the sick on whom they lay hands will recover."

An explicit statement of the supernatural power of God which will be manifest through his Church. The conditions are, of course, that it is for those who believe...God understands how difficult it is for us to believe and therefore he made provision of things we can experience which are supernatural and which help us to believe in the gospel. This is what is happening at the Ecumenical healing centre.

Whatever the purpose of healing and however it is conceived, all Christians see it as a result of God's will-full power, 'God's grace' in their words. The problem they then face is how to enable the sick person to receive this grace. One answer is to use prayer, to ask God for his grace either in very general terms, such as the intercessions made at the healing service, or for specific illnesses of specified individuals. Such prayer must however be selfless. To enable the will-full power of God to operate the person to be healed must give up their own will.

Dorothy Kerin in particular stressed this fact in her work:

Divine healing can only come when the soul has said: 'Lord it matters not to me whether I live or die except Thy will be done.' When the soul is thus attuned to the Divine will, the healing of the body must necessarily follow, provided it is God's will that it shall follow[15].

and

When we come to the Healing Service, our attitude should be one of hopeful expectancy and trust. We should leave the times and the means to God, and not make the mistake of trying to impose our own will, our own ways on Him. Our Lord knows best and we can safely leave the matter in his hands[15].

It is not just the patient who must will himself to have no will but also the healer if he or she wishes to act as a channel for the will of God. Thus Dorothy Kerin prayed before the laying on hands:

And now, O God, I give myself to Thee,
Empty me of all that is not of Thee;
Cleanse me of all unrighteousness,
And if it be Thy Will,
Take my hands and use them for Thy Glory,
Be it unto us according to Thy Will.

An idea expressed also at the Ecumenical healing centre by a trustee: 'You can't heal anybody...only the Lord can heal. You can be used as a channel of that grace but that grace can be withheld at any time,' and by a visiting speaker in a talk, 'The ministry is not a gift of particular people but one we can all act as channels for,' and by the chaplain in a sermon when he said 'we want to get rid of any thought of ourselves...(Jesus is) using us as his instruments'.

THE EXPERIENCE OF LOURDES EXAMINED

If Christians see healing as a manifestation of an omnipotent will-full God then it follows that such healing should be open to all people and in all places. Such in fact is the theological position. In practice however there are some people who seem to be more effective at healing than others. As one Christian healer expressed it to me: 'The theological view is "I don't do anything God does it through me" - humility. However the people involved in this are usually extremely brilliant characters. This contradicts the view that there must be nothing of yourself at all.'

Similarly there are some places which seem to be more effective than other places - shrines. Lourdes is one such shrine but there are many throughout the world[16]. Just as a magnifying glass can be used to focus the omnipresent rays of the sun to produce spectacular results, so Lourdes acts as a magnifying glass for the omnipresent power of God. To understand how Lourdes operates in this way it is necessary to understand the symbolism of the place. To do that we shall have to digress into sociological arguments about symbols and in particular look at the work of Mary Douglas (1970), Edward Leach (1976), and Victor Turner (1974a). Expressing their complicated arguments in simple terms we can say that they see power as being inherent in disorder. Mary Douglas summarizes this view when she says

> disorder by implication is unlimited, no pattern has been realised in it, but its potential for patterning is infinite. This is why though we seek to create order, we do not simply condemn disorder. We recognise that it is destructive to existing patterns; also that it has potentiality. It symbolizes both danger and power. (Douglas, 1970, p.114)

Disorder, thus argues Mary Douglas, is a symbol of danger and power. Taking this argument we can now return to Lourdes and look for disorder as a symbol of power. When we do this we find two sources of disorder at Lourdes. The first source of disorder, of power, is nature. Nature is disorderly, wild. Nature is outside the control of man and therefore potentially powerful. Looking for 'wild nature' at Lourdes we find it in the fact that Lourdes is sited in the 'wild' Pyrenees and has at its focus the 'natural' grotto. The second source of disorder, of power, occurs when there is a clash of symbols; then the categories of our thought overlap one with another to produce confusion. This is easiest to represent in a diagram (adapted from Leach, 1976, p.35):

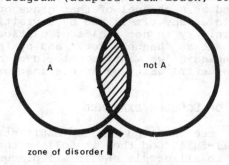

This boundary between the categories that men hold in their mind forms a zone of disorder. Turner (1974a, p.81) calls such an area a liminal state, from the Latin _limina_ meaning threshold. Pilgrimages, as Turner points out in his excellent article on the subject (1974b), are themselves liminal events. The pilgrimage is a time outside the normal conventions, demands and roles; as the old lady said, she went 'to get away from my telephone and my family - to recharge my batteries'. The pilgrimage is an experience of 'liminal disorder' when the normal social structure and hierarchy is laid on one side, the normal categories by which people relate to each other are forgotten and people interrelate as people and not as social roles, positions or statuses[17]. Thus in the terms of these sociological arguments about symbols the shrine of Lourdes may be viewed as a place of 'natural disorder' and the pilgrimage may be seen as a process of moving into and out of 'liminal disorder'. The pilgrimage to the shrine is a religious event which seeks to tap both 'natural disorder' and 'liminal disorder' at one and the same time. This is not the end of the argument, however, for more use can be made of the concept of 'liminality' than merely noting that a pilgrimage is a liminal event taking place in a gap between the normal everyday life of the pilgrims. We can note for example that the shrine grounds, the Domaine, lie on the margins of the town of Lourdes thus occupying a liminal position between the 'man-made' world of the town and the 'natural' world of the country. Similarly the grotto within the Domaine is a liminal place, the boundary where the world of God breaks through into the ordinary mundane world of man. It lies at the margin, the threshold, of this world and the other world. It is a channel for God's grace.

How though is this channel to be activated? How are people to gain access to this grace, this power? They do so through movement. The power is limited to the shrine and its immediate environs. For men to gain access to this power it is essential that they move from their homes to the shrine. Thus, through movement the power is brought into the service of man; movement is the trigger that releases the immense potential energy of the shrine. This point becomes even more obvious when one turns from looking at the movement to and from the shrine to looking at the movement within the shrine. The shrine, known as the 'Domaine', is an area of ground adjacent to the river. The Domaine is church property and is treated as a church in that smoking is not allowed, men are expected to wear jackets and women to cover their heads (although some relaxation of these restrictions has occurred recently). The Domaine is thus a sacred site set apart from the actual town of Lourdes. Within the Domaine there are a large number of buildings and natural features each of which have a part to play in either the running of the shrine as an institution or more importantly as aspects of the religious ritual which takes place in the shrine. Now, as we have seen, the shrine as a whole may be seen both as a 'natural' place in the foothills of the Pyrenees and as a 'liminal' place on the edge of town and of this world, but in addition there are internal divisions which are important if one is to understand events within the shrine. The simplest and most basic division is between the categories 'natural' and 'cultural'. The key point of the natural is the grotto and its spring. This is where Bernadette saw the visions of the immaculate conception; the point where the grotto is visible is also retained as a 'natural' area, known as the 'Prairie'. The key point of the 'cultural' is the basilica and the square in front of it. It is important to realise that the categories of 'natural' and 'cultural' are not the same as the division between 'sacred' and 'secular'. The whole Domaine, as pointed out above, is a sacred area containing places of various degrees of sacredness. However these cross-cut the division into nature and culture. Thus both the basilica and the grotto are sacred places but the first is a place of order, of culture and the second a place of disorder, of nature. Similarly the square is a site of order but it is not, except in so far as it is within the Domaine where all things are sacred, a sacred site. In fact the administrative offices are located around the square, as are such 'offices' as the toilets. The various distinctions between natural and cultural, sacred and secular, liminal disorder and natural disorder are all brought into play when the underground basilica is examined. This is a church - and therefore sacred. It is a building - and therefore cultural <u>but</u> it is built on the model of the inside of a whale[18] and it is built underground like the grotto - and is therefore natural. It is in this ambiguous, liminal place which is at one and the same time sacred, cultural and natural, that the crowning ritual of the Catholic faith, the high mass, is sung on Sundays - that most sacred day of the week. The ordinary basilica is not appropriate, for it is only sacred and cultural whilst the grotto is only sacred and natural[19].

Within this symbolic map the pilgrims move in procession. The point about movement is not just that it brings you physically into proximity with the place where the power lies but that it is fluid, changing. Categories are fixed, permanent, bounded. Movement is a means whereby the boundaries are broken open. By moving from one place to

another on the symbolic map the pilgrims enact a
metaphysical message. The two processions, the blessed
sacrament procession at four-thirty and the candlelight
procession at seven-thirty, each follow the same route and
take a similar form. Starting from the grotto the
participants in the procession line up behind a standard-
bearer who holds the standard of their group - by day a flag
and by night an illuminated sign. Tannoy announcements, in
several languages, exhort people to come together in the
square and show the unity of the Church, as the procession
forms. The procession then goes to the top of the Domaine
and down again to the square where the flags or standards
are taken up the steps at either side of the entrance to the
basilica. Apart from the standard-bearers the participants
all stand in the square in no particular order. In fact, at
the conclusion of the ceremony, when the host is taken into
the basilica, the participants leave the Domaine as
individuals[20] not as group members and the various groups
of pilgrims are inextricably tangled up, both literally and
figuratively, in their efforts to leave the Domaine through
the narrow exit. Even this short description makes it
obvious that the processions tap the power sited in the
grotto by moving from it to the square, moving from the
'natural' to the 'cultural'; from the site which is outside
man's control and therefore powerful to the site which is
man-made and where man has power[21]. The culmination of the
procession changes the classification of the participants as
differentiated groups into a mass of people who are
differentiated only into sick and others and who are seen to
express the unity of the Church. We can express this in a
simple diagram:

	Time 1		Time 2
Place	'Disorder' (natural grotto)	➡	'Order' (cultural square)
		Movement	
People	'Order' (group identity)	➡	'Disorder' (Church unity)

The diagram illustrates the almost algebraic transformation achieved by the processional movement. Movement
breaks down the categoric boundaries of group identity to
reintegrate men in the wider inclusive identity of members
of the Church. At the same time it breaks down the
boundaries of the grotto, the place of 'disorder' to tap the
awesome power situated here. It then controls this power by
taking the host, the most sacred object in the Christian
religion - the body of God - from the natural grotto to the
basilica. If 'disorder' is power, then power passes from the
place to the people, from the grotto to the church. It is no
accident that the culmination of the blessed sacrament
procession is not the communion service inside the basilica
but the point at which the host passes into the basilica,
sited above the grotto. The communion service is an epilogue

to a ritual completed.

As well as the key event of the processions there are other features of Lourdes which act, as it were, as sub-themes in the overall ritual score, sometimes becoming dominant and at other times fading away only to a murmur. One obvious sub-theme in the pilgrimage attended was the trip to the Cite de Secours. The participants, for the only time during the pilgrimage, wore 'disorderly' clothes - shorts, beach shirts, floppy hats - and took the sick outside the town into the 'wild' foothills of the Pyrenees and conducted a service in a 'natural' amphitheatre. The power of 'disorder' was being tapped. Disorder is also literally tapped by piping the spring which gushes up in the grotto into taps and into the baths. The baths are interesting because, as with the shrine as a whole, they contain both 'natural' disorder and 'liminal' disorder. The water is itself a symbol of the 'natural' being pure and unadulterated. It is also however a symbol of liminal disorder for in the baths it does not remain pure. As the sick are bathed in it, it rapidly becomes dirty and this fact was pointed out to me several times by informants during my day's service at the baths. Now dirt is a source of power because it is, in Mary Douglas's words (1970, p.48), 'matter out of place', i.e. a source of disorder. It is a liminal category. Another sub-theme is expressed in the tale of Bernadette, although it echoes in the procession. This is the theme of the Church as a cultural institution containing the power of 'natural disorder'. An examination of Bernadette's life, as expressed in the legends displayed in numerous books and several museums at Lourdes, shows her as a shepherd girl living in a semi-wild state amongst the hills around Lourdes. After seeing her visions she eventually became a nun, submitting herself to the order of the institutional Church. The 'myth' of Bernadette thus echoes and reiterates the message of Lourdes expressed in the processions and the baths. That message is that there is a mysterious source of power over which men have no control but that that source can be channelled by using the appropriate symbolic and ritual mechanisms.

CONCLUSION

Christian healing sees the source of healing as the immanent power of an omnipotent God: God's grace. To receive that power the afflicted persons must submit themselves entirely to God and remove all thought of self and self-will. In principle, this grace is available to all men at all places. In practice, channels for this grace are created. These channels may be people, in which case, like the afflicted, the channels must remove their own self-will to allow the will of God to flow through them. The channels may also be places, shrines, where it is believed God is especially present. Movement to and within shrines produces a channel for God's grace to flow to the afflicted[22].

NOTES

(1) Letter in the Ampleforth Hospitalite Newsletter of November 1978.
(2) There is an immense literature on Lourdes explaining its position in Catholicism. A good short description is provided in Turner and Turner (1978).
(3) Provided by the Bureau Medicale.
(4) Letter in the Ampleforth Hospitalite Newsletter of October 1976.
(5) A pseudonym, as is Marie.
(6) Taken from The Church of Christ the Healer, pamphlet.
(7) The information in this section about the routine of Burrswood comes from a visit and an interview with Dr Cuming, who was the warden at the time of my visit (1976). He has now retired and the routine may have changed.
(8) The name of the centre has been withheld.
(9) Taken from the AGM report of the centre in 1975.
(10) I analysed these by sex (this was possible because with the exception of two cases, where surnames were used, only Christian names were read out). There were 58 males, 116 females and 10 I was not able to classify making a total of 184 people for whom intercession was made.
(11) A pseudonym.
(12) A trustee of the centre.
(13) A speaker at the centre.
(14) From On What Should a Doctor Base His Decisions? by Dr E. Aubert MD, undated pamphlet.
(15) From Dorothy Kerin and Divine Healing, undated pamphlet.
(16) In addition to Lourdes I've visited St Joseph's Oratory, Montreal; the Virgin of Guadalupe in Mexico City and Walsingham in Norfolk. For descriptions of many shrines see Turner and Turner (1978).
(17) Turner calls such a state communitas and distinguishes between normative, existential and ideological forms (Turner, 1974a). These distinctions are not necessary for the present argument so will not be pursued.
(18) This was reported to me several times by different people. Its truth or falsity as a matter of historic fact is immaterial to the argument which is concerned with mytho-logical truth.
(19) Sheer numbers may have something to do with this but it would be possible to accommodate the same vast numbers on the Prairie as throng the underground basilica.
(20) The exception of this is that each brancadier pulls a sick person out in a carriage.
(21) It may be significant that the centre of most French towns is known as a place, (square) i.e. the heart of the cultural in contrast to the natural in ordinary life has the same name as the heart of the cultural at Lourdes.
(22) Another way in which a bridge between this world and the other world may be made is through sacrifice (see e.g. Leach, 1976). I have not dealt with the problem of sacrifice here because it did not arise in any healing I observed.

4 Radiesthesia

When people cut their hair or nails in some African societies they are very careful to collect all the clippings. This is not an obsessive concern with tidiness but a fear that others, gaining possession of these fragments, might gain power over the owner through witchcraft. Nail parings, hair, sputum or blood provide the witch or sorcerer with a representation of his victim, a representation upon which he can bring to bear his magical powers. Now such objects are also important to the practice of the healers examined in this chapter. Blood spots on blotting paper are carried by the British postman to members of the Psionic Medical Society and to other radionic practitioners. Yet these healers, far from seeing themselves engaged in witchcraft, do not even see it as a religious act. Unlike all the healers looked at so far in this book they are not concerned with religious or magical forces. Rather they claim to be acting scientifically, that the force they utilise is not religious but natural. It is the force which moves a pendulum or a dowsing rod in the hands of a person with a 'radiesthetic' faculty - the ability to dowse. They are engaged in medical dowsing. Radiesthesia they claim, is a scientific technique and the force which moves the pendulum is a natural force not a supernatural one and consequently it is open to precise scientific investigation and measurement. To examine this claim it will be necessary to define what is meant by science. Before doing this, however, we need to look at the theory and practice of radionics in some detail, a detail provided by examining three users of radiesthesia: psionic medicine, radionics and cymatics.

PSIONIC MEDICINE

The practice of psionic medicine is explained in one of the publications of the psionic medical society:

> Psionic diagnosis and treatment is simple in concept
> and it has been found that in the hands of an expert
> it gives reliable information and results, largely

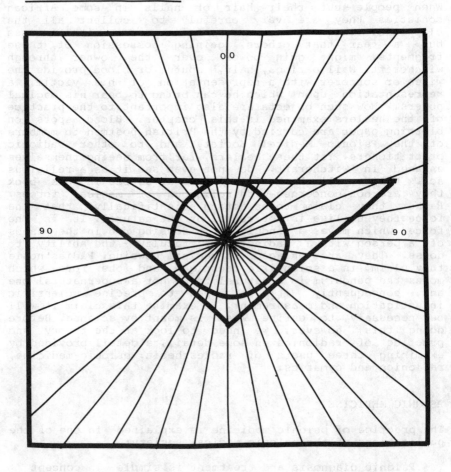

unobtainable by ordinary diagnostic and therapeutic means.

The concept on which it is based is: Health is a state of balance and harmony on all planes; or, in radiesthetic terms - a balanced, harmonious behaviour of energy patterns constitutes health. Any loss of balance, however slight, constitutes ill-health; gross and chronic imbalance is disease.

If health is now represented as 0, or zero, on a diagnostic chart or rule, then ill-health and disease are represented by a deviation from the norm (zero) by a plus or minus reading, the pendulum registering this in degrees on the chart.

This concept is represented in a geometric diagram or chart consisting of a circle, a triangle, and a square, and is constituted as follows: the triangle has a base-line of 12 inches, and the apex (pointing downwards) is 5 inches from the base-line. The circle inside the triangle has a diameter of 4 inches, just touching the base-line at its midpoint, so the centre of the circle is 2 inches from the base-line and is also at the centre of the square. The circle is divided into lines radiating at 10-degree intervals left and right of the mid-perpendicular line, which is the zero line. The lines are extended to the edges of the square, 14x14 inches, which encloses the triangle and the circle. These measurements and angles are critical.

The technique both of diagnosis and treatment, when using this diagram, is based on the establishment of an equilibrium of forces between three factors: the patient's witness, usually a blood spot (but this can be hair or a saliva or urine specimen), which is placed in the right hand corner of the triangle; the diagnostic witness or witnesses placed in the left-hand corner; and the radiesthetically indicating remedies, usually homoeopathic, are placed in the apex of the triangle. These together should establish a state of dynamic balance, registering as zero on the diagnostic pattern, and recorded by the pendulum swinging up and down the zero line.

This technique can be used for the resolution of most medical problems, as by its means it is possible to arrive at the fundamental causal factors lying at the root of the state of ill-health, and equally to determine the exact treatment required to eliminate them, and thus enable the patient's own inner vital healing resources to function once the inhibiting factor is removed. Provided, of course, that no irreversible changes have occurred in vital tissues or organs, though even in these cases it is often found that the patient can be made more comfortable and more amenable to symptomatic treatment.

It must be admitted that psionic medicine depends on the right and efficient functioning of a supersensible sense - the radiesthetic faculty - and it may be justly queried as to what reliance can be placed on a psychic gift of this nature[1].

This explanation of the practice was expanded on in an interview with Aubrey Westlake, then the vice-president of the Psionic Medical Society, when I asked him what he did when a patient came to see him.

Usually they've had all sorts of other treatments. What I do is to take an exhaustive history...back to grandparents, everything they've had the matter with them in their lives. Having got that, after a time you can more or less tell what you're likely to find radiesthetically. Then you take a blood spot, or a hair specimen, or saliva or urine. You then test that according to the radiesthetic technique. You may not get the causal factors to start with; it's like an archaeological excavation. You start off with the indicated treatment.

You're dealing with something that isn't material or physical. What is the treatment appropriate for that? It is homoeopathy[2] because after the twelfth potency you can prove mathematically there isn't any matter there. As you know it goes on to 30, 100, 1,000, 10,000 and so on. What have we got? Because they're effective...What in fact happens, the classic method of potentisation is de-materialisation. You're getting rid of the matter, you're liberating the vital essence of the drug you are using. In the very high potencies you've practically got the drug in its essence, in its archetypal form...that's what we usually use. Radiesthetically controlled homoeopathy. The pendulum decides which. It will both give you what it is you wanted and the potency.

The indicated treatment might last a fortnight. You say, 'You report and we'll do a check-up to see what you want.' Now one of the things people don't understand...you hardly ever give the same treatment twice. The reason is quite obvious: if the medicine has had any effect it alters the pattern. Therefore you've got to have a different prescription next time. So you go on gradually clearing them...until their readings are zero, or near zero.

The influence of homoeopathy upon the practice of Dr Westlake is not only shown in the use of homoeopathic medicines, it is also demonstrated by his insistence that treatment is of the individual not the disease.

Since it is a basic tenet of homoeopathy that the

treatment is related to the individual and not merely
to the ailment, the prescription is essentially
dependent on an understanding of the patient[3].

and

Treatment is entirely individual and consists
essentially in stimulating and co-operating with the
healing force of the body[4].

thus

the aim of treatment is in fact to remove the causes
of lowered vitality which lead to disease
susceptibility[4].

And the influence of homoeopathy is also shown in the
homoeopathic notion of miasm which Dr Westlake explained in
these terms:

Hahnemnann in the last twelve years of his long life
devoted it to trying to discover why it was patients
he had treated homoeopathically, and rightly, then
relapsed. He was concerned with this question of
chronic disease and he finally elaborated the idea
there was what he called a miasmic factor, which
unless you got rid of it you would never cure the
patient. For example, suppose your great-grandmother
had tuberculosis...it will then be passed down as
what we call a miasmic condition and this is
responsible for a lot of things ordinary medicine
can't deal with, like migraines, allergies, sinus
trouble...[3].

The practitioners of psionic medicine are few in number -
102 paid-up members in 1976 according to the treasurer's
report. However, this small membership is in part a product
of the deliberate exclusivity of the Psionic Medical Society
which restricts full membership to qualified medical and
dental practitioners although allowing others to join as
associate members:

The Society originated with Dr Guyon Richards, who
gathered around him a distinguished group of doctors,
and they formed the Medical Society for the Study of
Radiesthesia...Guyon Richards died in 1946; five
other distinguished members died in the next five
years, so the original group was almost wiped out.
Only a few were left, one being Dr George Laurence,
and he proceeded to carry on the work and make it
into something that could be taught. He produced what
we call the science part of it and he coined the word
psionic...About five years ago we formed the Psionic
Medical Society[3].

RADIONICS

The members of the Psionic Medical Society use a simple
pendulum and chart to diagnose but there are some users of
the dowsing or radiesthetic faculty who use instead a black
box. These boxes were originally developed by Dr Drown in
America and are distributed in Britain through a
professional organisation, the Radionics Association, and
through a business organisation, Delawarr Laboratories. The
boxes act as a sort of calibrated pendulum to tap the
radiesthetic force:

> Basic to radionic theory and practice is the concept
> that man and all life-forms share a common ground in
> that they are submerged in the electro-magnetic
> energy field of the Earth; and further that each
> life-form has its own electro-magnetic field which,
> if sufficiently disturbed, will ultimately result in
> disease of the organism.

> Accepting that 'All is Energy', Radionics sees
> organs, diseases and remedies as having their own
> particular frequency or vibration. These factors can
> be expressed in numerical values and are known in
> radionics as 'Rates'.

> The radionic practitioner in making his analysis
> utilizes the principle of dowsing by applying his
> faculties of extra-sensory perception (ESP) to the
> problem of detecting disease in much the same way as
> the dowser detects the location of water, oil or
> mineral deposits...
> ...the standard practice when a radionic practitioner
> is consulted is for the patient to send the
> practitioner a blood spot or hair sample accompanied
> by a case history and a full description of symptoms.
> In order to make an analysis the practitioner places
> the patient's sample on his radionic instrument, then
> attunes his mind to the patient and adjusts his
> instrument in a way which is analogous to the
> adjustment or tuning, of a radio to receive a distant
> transmission[4].

The normal instrument, which is primarily designed for
diagnosis, is contained in a black suitcase. The suitcase is
opened so that the lid lies to the left. The lid of the
suitcase contains a space for a large card. There is also a
bar which can be slid up or down over the card. The base of
the case contains two metal cups at the far end and thirteen
calibrated knobs. At the end nearest the user there is a
rubber membrane[5]. The full diagnostic procedure consists
of placing in the lid a card for the whole body which lists
the various organs and symptoms. The specimen is placed, in
its envelope, in one of the cups (left for male, right for
female). The bar is then moved down the card with the left
hand while the right strokes the membrane. When the membrane
becomes 'sticky' it means the bar is above the diseased

organ or system. Next to the list of organs and systems on the card is a set of 'rates' (precalculated by the instrument makers). The dials on the far end of the box are then set to these rates and another card inserted in the lid which is more specific, in that it lists parts of organs and systems. The procedure is repeated with greater and greater specificity. In fact the patient usually supplies the practitioner with a set of symptoms. A practitioner justified this practice to me by pointing out that to fully carry out a diagnosis using an instrument would take months and that the person coming for help for his affliction does, after all, want to get rid of his pain as soon as possible. The radionic practitioner is thus morally obliged to find the cause of the affliction as quickly as possible to enable treatment to take place, and this process is speeded up if the radionic practitioner knows which cards he should use in the machine.

When the radionic analysis is complete and the practitioner has accurately ascertained the major causative factors of the patient's illness, he determines what form of treatment is required by the patient to remove those factors. As all pathological states and their causes have their own particular frequency or vibration, he selects those Rates which will offset the imbalance or disease in the patient's system. These Rates are projected or transmitted by the practitioner to the patient by means of a radionic treatment instrument, once again using the blood spot or hair sample as a link. Some practitioners use, as an adjunct to the healing influence of the Rate, homoeopathic, Bach (flower) or other similar remedies. These are placed on the instrument in proximity to the patient's sample[4].

Anyone can be taught to use the instrument and the majority of the population appear to have the radiesthetic faculty to some degree. However, to use the instrument properly requires not just a radiesthetic faculty but also knowledge of the physiology of the human body so that readings of the instrument can be correctly interpreted. For its practitioners radionics is thus not mysterious but simply hard work.

The demand for treatment using radiesthesia is constant and Delawarr Laboratories, for example, had 189 treatment instruments in operation when I visited them, coping with 250 people (some people sharing a treatment instrument). In addition at certain times of the year they treat two stables of racehorses as well as the occasional pet animal.

CYMATICS

Many radionic practitioners never see their patients, relying on the postal service to bring the specimens upon which they can operate. In contrast, the practitioner of cymatic medicine requires the physical presence of a patient in treatment for he 'injects' his patients with sound.

The village where the practitioner I saw had his clinic was straight out of a 1930s Hollywood film set in the English countryside. One expected a border collie to pad round the corner any minute. Even the pub had an uneven roof-ridge and roses around the door, giving an impression of cardboard cut-outs. The clinic was a Victorian house on the opposite side of the road to the pub, hidden behind a wall and some trees. Three small brass plaques on the door announced in capital letters: John Mark Hartley LBCP, MSEI (London), Osteopath, homoeopath, ray and electro-therapist, and Anne Hartley MAB TH, radionic consultant[6].

Inside it was large and chillingly damp. It was also dark and somewhat gloomy - heavy clouds overhead making the day very dark. The atmosphere was not, however, the menacing one that the description of the house may have suggested. Rather it was the sort of atmosphere that one gets at village fetes that are forced into the church hall because of bad weather, an atmosphere of bustling busyness dominated by middle-aged ladies in tweed dresses.

I was shown through into a large room overlooking the side garden and there left to wander around looking at the books, ornaments, photographs and certificates that were on all walls and surfaces. The room wasn't cluttered but it was occupied by objects, much like a country vicar's study. There, in time, I interviewed John Hartley. He, like the village, exuded an air of artificiality but here too the impression was wrong, his bouncy energy and his commitment to what he is doing came over as very real. He became involved in healing because

> my mother was in it to begin with and I was going to take up ordinary medicine...but after a short space of time I soon found that just wasn't my cup of tea. I wanted to be more involved with the patient rather than sitting behind a desk writing out prescriptions-...so I broke off from that, went into osteopathy. I studied homoeopathy, and then ultimately I went to Germany to study because someone was doing specialised work there. That's how I came into what we term cymatics - the use of sound.

To help him in this work he has five staff, some part-time, and his wife.

After the interview I was taken on a tour of the house. We started at the front of the house. To the right as one enters through the front door there is an office with a receptionist, to the left a door leads into a room partitioned off into six cubicles by boarding which doesn't reach to the high ceiling. Curtains form the front of each cubicle. Inside each there is a bed and the treatment machine which looks like an old-fashioned piece of medical equipment with a cassette tape deck on it. After glancing at the lights above the door through which we entered the room (red for female, blue for male) which signify which cubicles are occupied. John Hartley took me into several of the cubicles. He was wearing a white coat and carrying a clipboard. He went in and out of each cubicle rapidly, chatting briefly to the clients. The impression generated was that of a busy doctor on ward rounds. His assistants, who are nurses, do the actual treatment which in the main consists of placing pads, connected by wires to the treatment machine, onto the patients. The patients lie on the beds in their underwear under bright heat lamps which keep them warm. The pads were moved from place to place on the patients' bodies.

The pads and the treatment machine form the major treatment at this healing centre - namely sound therapy. There are, however, other modes of treatment used: for patients with arthritis a vibrator and massage is used and for patients with emotional problems colour therapy is used.

John Hartley explained his practice to me in interview: When the patient arrives 'they come in, they go to the front office. She just takes their name and address and just a general sort of condition. She doesn't interview them. Then she puts them into either one of the cubicles and then she calls me. I go and interview the patient, get the details and then assess the treatment'.

The details are recorded on a sheet of paper:

> We have a space on the top in which we take down as near as possible exactly what the patient says. Not our terminology of it because I think this confuses the issue. They tell us what they feel or what is the trouble, how they see it, how they view it. Then there are various questions we ask them such as what treatments they've had previously, whether they've been sent by their general practitioner, or whether they've come of their own accord, whether they're on drug therapy or any medication of any kind. Then, finally...we examine the case and put our diagnosis on it.

> The pattern's changing now. In the earlier days everyone had been to their doctor and their hospital and found no relief and then we got them...at the tail-end. (But) our clinic has been here so long now we're getting people that haven't even been to their doctor or hospital (but) come in and start treatment right away. In these cases of course we get a greater measure of success because we treat them early...But the other cases...sometimes years they've been under treatment which has given no benefit whatsoever... Although you can very often improve or ease these conditions, you can't clear them up. They're of too long standing.

Of the diseases he deals with

the majority, the biggest percentage of them is
muscular disorders - arthritis, rheumatoid fibrositis
- we're in that kind of area where people are working
on farms, growers, horticulturists. Therefore, a
great percentage of our cases are arthritis, spinal
trouble, bone disorder.

Treatment is decided in accordance with the
condition itself, but we're finding that cymatics is
taking over more and more from the ordinary sort of
treatments.

The theory behind cymatic practice is that

If you take a sounding off an ordinary muscle
structure you'll find it produces a signal...The whole
muscle is in a state of movement fluctuation;
therefore it produces a signal. Now if there's an
arthritic condition within that structure the signal
will be slightly different.
What we do - we use the term 'inject' but this is
rather confusing because we don't use a hypodermic
needle - is use an applicator which projects the
sound in. So we inject the sound of a normal healthy
signal. We put the healthy signal into where there is
a variation and invariably that variation will re-
align itself...nature is very prone with even a small
amount of assistance to return to the normal rather
than stay in the abnormal. So what we do is to inject
into the area the normal signal; the muscle responds
to it, it becomes more relaxed...it beats in
pulsation and union with the signal that's going in
and invariably you can manipulate...create deep
massage because it's more relaxed...In some cases the
abnormality will revert to the normal purely...-
because you've injected the signal.

The normal signal is obtained in two ways

One is orthodox and one is unorthodox. The orthodox
is to put an applicator onto the area of muscle, a
very delicate microphone in a soundproof room, then
you can pick off that signal. Then you can record it,
and amplify it, and put it onto tape. You can then
throw it up onto a graph and see it or put it onto a
sound producing thing...

We can do it by a radionic technique. If you set up
a computer of multi-oscillations and someone who has
a radionic technique either uses a detector pad or
the pendulum and the other person operates the signal
on the generator by turning slowly the person
produces a 'stick'. Then you hold it at that point,
then you try the next one and the next one and so on,

until you build up your signal. Then you compute these and record them and you will get the precise picture. This is without touching the patient.

To achieve this you can use a hair specimen or the patient can be present - there's no hard and fast rule.

In the case of muscles, bones, nerve fibres, there is a kind of norm which applies to all human beings. This doesn't apply when it comes to internal organs or other structures of the body. Therefore cymatics can't be done in that simplified way if you want to treat the kidney or heart or intestinal wall because these vary with size, shape, age, sex. All sorts of things make a difference. But muscle structure, nerve fibre, bone conditions - arthritis, rheumatoid arthritis, rheumatism, fibrositis, muscular injuries, bone conditions, bone abnormalities - are things which can be treated clinically by nurses. All these various ones are in the rack...all these reels of magnetic tapes are marked. All the nurses do is take it out and put it into the instrument and then apply it to the area which is written on the case sheet. But if you have a condition (this is the field of research we are moving into now) where you have to treat an abnormality within organs then an organ produces a mass harmonic because there are various signals within that organ in accordance with its size and shape as well as its construction...What we are doing gradually is taking a signal from the abnormality and assessing it against a norm pattern. In other words you put it onto a graph, put one graph over the other and see where the abnormalities are.

The length of treatment, as with the mode of treatment,

depends on condition, approximately half an hour...Every patient is an individual. It's dealt with, talked to, treated...if we came under the National Health the doctor would say 'Go to Woodstock Hall, Woodstock Hall, Woodstock Hall' with the consequent result that we would be cluttered up with patients who we wouldn't be able to treat. We'd just be overwhelmed. We've got more than we can cope with comfortably now...forty, fifty, sixty a day...we manage somehow...and if someone rings up because they're in trouble we always keep an emergency treatment room clear.

SCIENCE OR MAGIC?

Radiesthesia along with orthodox medicine claims to be scientific. A superficial glance at their pamphlets and books would seem to confirm this claim. The language they use and the theory they generate to explain disease have all the characteristics of science:

> Basic to radionic theory and practice is the concept
> that all life-forms share a common ground in that
> they are submerged in the electro-magnetic field of
> the earth; and further, that each life-form has its
> own electro-magnetic field, which, if sufficiently
> disturbed, will ultimately result in disease of the
> organism[4].

That they have not been able to measure these fields or
fully explain them is no bar to their theory being accepted
as scientific. Gravity too can only be measured by its
effects and is not fully explained. It is when one turns to
their method of diagnosis that doubts about the scientific
nature of their enterprise begin to arise. They diagnose
using the faculty of dowsing, and dowsing is not a
scientific procedure but the operation of a psychic gift as
they themselves state: 'It must be admitted that psionic
medicine depends on the right and efficient functioning of a
supersensible sense - the radiesthetic faculty - and it may
justly be queried as to what reliance can be placed on a
psychic gift of this nature'[1].

The operation of such a gift means that diagnosis is
always uncertain. This in turn means that when a patient
fails to recover the failure of the treatment can be blamed
on a misdiagnosis, and hence the general theory remains
unchallenged. It is important to note however that this is
not a characteristic peculiar to radionic diagnosis. The
diagnostic procedure in orthodox medicine is also considered
to be an art rather than a science, with similar
consequences[7].

Further doubts arise when one looks at their method of
treatment. In their diagnosis they utilise 'witnesses',
samples of blood, hair, or nail parings, as does orthodox
medicine when it takes blood samples and asks for a urine
specimen. However orthodox medicine does not take the part
to represent the whole person, and more importantly it does
not try to treat the whole person by treating the sample.
This is what radionic treatment does for it claims that by
changing the shape of the energy field around a specimen it
thus changes the shape of the energy field around the
individual from whom the specimen was taken. This sounds
much more like sorcery than science. The 'witnesses' or
'specimens' are similar to those used by sorcerers: hair,
nails, sputum, urine and blood. All of these it has been
argued have symbolic meaning in addition to their
convenience as easily portable representations of an
individual. Douglas (1973) argues that hair, nails, and
sputum are all parts of an individual that are on the body
boundary. As such they are potentially powerful being
liminal objects that are both of the individual and yet not
of him. They are difficult to categorise and therefore
potentially capable of creating new categorical forms. They
are thus powerful and dangerous. Blood can also be described

in this manner but is perhaps more appropriately dealt with as a symbol expressing the essential essence of a person, their identity. We talk of 'blood relations' and use phrases such as 'blood is thicker than water' to express our belief that blood is a powerful symbol of identity. As Turner (1974c) points out, it is also a fundamental physiological symbol intimately associated with birth and life. It is therefore very appropriate that those wishing for a change in life, a change from being sick to being healthy should give blood as their 'witness'. Radionic therapists appear to be committing the 'sorcerer's error' (Leach, 1976) in which a part is taken to represent the whole, and action upon this symbolic representation is presumed to effect change in the whole by sympathetic magic. One of the features of such sorcery is that distance is no bar to its action, which radionic practice also claims: 'As the treatment is not physical the distance by which the practitioner and the patient are separated is quite immaterial'[8].

Doubts about the scientific nature of radionic diagnosis and therapy force one to look at what is implied by the notion of science. What underlies our judgement of radionics as scientific, magical or religious is a view which sees science and religion as distinguished from each other by different applications of the concept of 'will'. Science is a mode of understanding and a procedure which stresses the active will of man. The cosmology of science explains events in terms of abstract forces which have no will, natural forces acting blindly without intent. The procedure science has adopted to comprehend these forces is that of the experiment. In the experiment the scientist seeks to bring under his control all the variables involved so that he can manipulate them and get answers to his questions about the manner in which abstract will-less forces work. Science stresses the objectivity of this approach, its independence of the individual scientist. Any man following the same procedures will get the same answers because natural forces, being will-less, are constant in their action. Furthermore, the understanding that is achieved through an experiment is communicable to all.

Religion, in contrast, is a mode of understanding and a procedure which stresses the passive will of man[9]. The cosmology of religion explains events in terms of personalised forces which have will and act with intent and purpose. The procedure of religion through which one 'comprehends' these forces is typically that of ritual. Through ritual man seeks to produce a state in which the forces work on himself and on nature. He can prepare by cleansing himself of 'self' so as to be open to the forces, but he cannot ensure he will gain comprehension. It is the will of the forces he is addressing and not his own will that decide if he gains comprehension. Purity and spirituality may help but ultimately the comprehension comes as a gift from the will of the forces, a charism, a grace of God. Not all individuals receive this grace and nor is it communicable to others. Thus the same procedures will not always produce the same results; there is consequently an element of uncertainty of outcome built into religious procedures which contrasts sharply with the certainty of outcome of scientific procedures. Religious understanding is not gained but granted; scientific understanding is achieved.

An extension of this distinction in terms of will also serves to delineate magic and technology from each other and from religion. Both magic and technology are attempts to impose man's will on events. However, magic seeks to control forces that have will (spirits, demons) whereas technology seeks to control will-less forces. For both magic and technology there is an element of uncertainty in the outcome of attempts at control. To understand the world science abstracts and simplifies using a mode of expression that is most certain, logic and mathematics, wherever possible. However the application of science to control events, technology, has to deal not with an abstract but a real world and this means ambiguities and uncertainties creep back in. The technologist cannot know all the features of the real world nor can he control them all. If the scientist can be compared to the architect drawing up plans, the technologist is the builder who has to execute those plans and cope with the vagaries of materials, labour and weather. The outcome of magic, too, is uncertain because the forces it deals with have will and may seek to assert their will over the magician. Thus in both magic and technology there is an attempt to eliminate uncertainty by the precision of the procedures used: 'Magic is surrounded by strict conditions: exact remembrance of a spell, unimpeachable performance of the rite, unswerving adherence to the taboos and observances' (Malinowski, 1954, p.85).

In both practices, the understanding of the means of imposing one's will comes through knowledge. To be a technologist or to be a magician requires study and dedication - unlike religious understanding it is not a gift.

Let us now turn back to radionics and look once again at their explanation of disease. They see disease as caused by a disharmony in a material force or by a shadow in the etheric or spiritual realm, a 'miasm' (Reyner et al., 1974). Now explanations of disease appear to locate the causes of it in three types of force: spiritual, material and social. If we now classify these forces against their 'will' an interesting pattern emerges:

Table 2 Forces' Will

Type of force	Will-full	Will-less
Spiritual	1. Demons spirits	2. Miasms (radionic theory)
Material	3. -	4. Germs, Azande witches[10] disharmony (radionic theory)
Social	5. -	6. Psychosomatic disease

The problems for the sociologist trying to classify radionic practitioners is now apparent. In terms of a crude criteria of science which sees it as dealing only with the material world, their insistence on a spiritual world precludes them from the claim to be scientific. If however we define science in the terms I have used above, as the explanation of events in terms of abstract forces possessing no will, then they must be granted a scientific status. So, it is not just in terms of how they explain disease that radionic practitioners may be seen as scientific (after all, their use of scientific terminology may hide an unscientific mode of thought and so be merely 'scientism'), but also in terms of what they are explaining.

Explanation of disease is not however the only aspect of a healing practice, nor is it necessarily the most important part. Diagnosis is a procedure of asking questions. Now is this procedure as used in radionics a scientific procedure, a religious procedure, a medical procedure or a technical procedure? It has many of the characteristics of a technical or magical procedure. For example, it requires of its practitioners a knowledge base.

In addition there is an insistence on precision. The instructions for constructing a psionic diagnostic chart end with the words 'These measurements and angles are critical' and radionic practitioners try to control the construction of their black boxes so that they are made exactly to their specifications. Finally almost everyone can be taught to diagnose. It would thus appear that radionic diagnosis is a technical skill not tied to any particular individual. However it is also asserted that the essence of radionic diagnosis is a 'psychic gift' which has very uncertain outcomes, such that replication is to be avoided: Reyner and his associates (Reyner et al., 1974) in their book on psionic medicine argue that a person beginning to use dowsing must avoid repeating the dowsing procedure. Such repetition is considered by them to fog the dowsing faculty, and an individual who wants a reliable answer is advised to have a clear mind and a precise question rather than seek reliability through replication.

87

From this evidence radionics appears to be a religious procedure: the individual gives up his will to the dowsing force, the pendulum moves independent of his volition. On the other hand the force that moves the pendulum is will-less. Will-less forces lie in the domain of science, not religion. As with their explanation of disease, so too with their procedures of diagnosis, radionic practitioners lie ambiguously between science and technology on the one hand and religion and magic on the other.

The picture becomes even more confused when we turn finally to the therapy; their method of treatment seems on superficial examination to be a clear case of magic. Their explanation of their therapy is that healing is a consequence of a change in an abstract will-less force. This explanation, as I have already argued, is not a religious explanation because it talks of will-less forces, albeit spiritual will-less forces. Nor is their actual therapy religious or magical. Religious therapy requires of healer or patient, or both, that they open themselves to a spiritual power and lose their will. In fact many religious healers tell of their own gift coming to them only after they have stopped trying to assert their own will and bowed to the will of God[11]. Radionic therapy on the other hand is seen as a manipulation of an abstract will-less force, a technological act rather than a religious or a magical one. A technician can be used to implement radionic treatment, it does not require a person who has a radiesthetic faculty, only a person who can follow clear instructions given by someone with the faculty.

CONCLUSION

A superficial examination of radionics would place it clearly in the realm of sorcery rather than science. It talks of an unmanifest reality, an etheric realm (Reyner, 1974), utilises the parts of people that witches used and use - their nails, hair, urine, sputum and blood - and it treats those parts as though they were the whole person, expecting a change in the part to produce a change in the whole. In addition its therapy claims to act at a distance, and its diagnosis relies on a psychic gift which is uncertain in its outcome but which requires precision in its execution.

However when one examines it more closely difficulties in this simple classification begin to appear. The forces it talks of are blind, they are not the will-full forces of religion and magic but the will-less forces of science. Its diagnosis requires the individual to give up his will, but he does so not to a will-full force but to a will-less one. Also, diagnosis requires knowledge and precision, which are both characteristics of magic and technology rather than religion, and although the ability to dowse is a gift it appears to be a gift we all possess, and so everyone can be taught to diagnose. Finally, its therapy is a technical act, not a religious or magical one. It requires no special powers on the part of the operator, only an obedience to instructions.

Radionics is thus a healing method that seems to be both scientific and spiritual. This presents problems for the sociologist trying to analyse and classify the activities and theories of radionic practitioners. For practitioners, however, it means that they can appeal to two publics: the scientific and the spiritual. A stress on the scientific aspects of their practice attracts those with scientific interests. A stress on the spiritual aspects attracts those with spiritual interests. The ambiguity is thus not a weakness but a strength because it enables radionics to appeal to a much wider audience than would be possible if it were wholly scientific or wholly spiritual.

NOTES

(1) From 'An Outline of Psionic Medicine', reprinted from the Journal of the Psionic Medical Society, autumn 1973.
(2) Homoeopathy is a theory and practice of therapy initiated by Hahnemann, a German physician, in the late eighteenth century. Homoeopathic remedies are applied to a patient to produce similar symptoms to those he is suffering from. The more severe the symptoms the weaker the dose of the drug given. To weaken a drug it is diluted by being mixed with water or alcohol (or both). A dilution of one measure of a drug to nine measures of fluid is called the first potency. The twelfth potency is one part in a billion.
(3) From the interview with Dr Westlake.
(4) From An Introduction to Radionics (1973), pamphlet of the Radionic Association.
(5) A picture of a radionic diagnostic instrument is shown on pp.124 and 125 of Kingston (1975) where he describes Delawarr Laboratories.
(6) The names are pseudonyms.
(7) For an excellent discussion of this point in orthodox medicine see Millman (1977).
(8) From A Simple Outline of Radionic Treatment, undated pamphlet of the Radionic Association.
(9) See the discussion in the previous chapter and also see Lienhardt's (1961), concept of passiones.
(10) The Azande, according to Evans-Pritchard (1937), see their witches as being witches because of a witch organ. This is a biological entity which is inherited. It is therefore not under the control of the witch; he does not will his witchcraft. Thus following their cosmology strictly we are here dealing with a material will-less force. In practice the Azande appear to presume will on the part of the witch sometimes and are not clear on this point.
(11) See for example the Filipino healer described in the first chapter. See also Gelfland (1964) and Frankenberg and Leeson (1976).

5 'Eastern' healers

HOSPITAL

Visitors

1. Please announce yourself.
2. Please do not bring articles of food or drink without medical consent. It tempts patients to disrupt diets.
3. Patients have been begged to refrain from normal worrying activities and very often advised to isolate themselves in the first few days.

Please help them and us in this respect.
Thank you.

This notice, with a small hand-bell standing next to it, was at the foot of the stairs in the Ramana Health Centre[1]. Although only a few miles down the road from White Eagle Lodge (see p.32) it is a very different place. Without explicit directions I would never have found it in spite of the fact that it is only a short distance from the main London to Portsmouth road, for it is hidden away down country lanes. The building is an old one, possibly thirteenth century, but was obviously renovated in Victorian times to become a modest manor, set in extensive wooded grounds. Inside it has wood-panelled walls and wooden floors. The interior is very like Burrswood except it is not so well cared for, nor so well polished, and lacks the flowers and the brightness of Burrswood. The largest room in the building is the 'library', furnished with large settees and armchairs, which serves as a room for relaxation as well as being the chapel; an apse at one end has within it an altar with a statue of Buddha and two crosses on it and a stained-glass window behind. The majority of the other rooms are private rooms for patients but there are also rooms equipped for hydrotherapy, in which patients bathe to raise their temperature and sweat out impurities, an x-ray room, and a homoeopathic dispensary in which radionic diagnosis can be undertaken.

The hope of the director, Dr Sharma, is to extend the facilities to give complete coverage:

> The Ramana Health Centre has been established to service people in need of all forms of alternative medicine, with homoeopathy as the hub and including osteopathy, Alexander technique, Chinese medicine, ayurvedic medicine, etc...When complete the hospital will consist of all departments: mother and baby unit, general medical unit, surgical and out-patient unit, lecturing and training facilities[2].

A qualified medical doctor, Dr Sharma was cured of a paralysis of the spine by homoeopathy, which turned his interest to alternative therapies. His study and use of them persuaded him that they all contained unsolved problems and omissions. In addition, when his patients were seriously ill they were taken into orthodox hospitals and could not continue their unorthodox treatment. So he set up the Ramana Health Foundation to run Ludshott Manor Hospital as the Ramana Health Centre, a place where orthodox and unorthodox treatment methods could be practised under supervision of qualified medical practitioners: 'The purpose of Ludshott is to make sure soberness exists. We want the orthodox to understand the unorthodox and we want to ensure the unorthodox does not run into quackery. My intention was to rescue alternative medicine from quackery by setting up a proving place[3]'.

The philosophy underlying the treatment at Ludshott is that 'illness is not something of which one need be afraid, rather it is an evolution. It is not an isolated event, but invariably the result of the person's whole way of living[2]'. Up to twenty patients can be accommodated at the hospital. However, it is not full; few doctors other than the director refer their patients there. Those patients who do arrive are met by a nurse who introduces them to the others in the hospital and talks to them about how they'll be treated:

> We put most people on a fast at the beginning. I prepare them for frustrations. They're mainly put on a three-day cut yourself off trip. No books are allowed except the Bible and (Dr Sharma's) book - no telephone, papers, television, radio. They often also fast for the three days, although people are usually put on a day's fast[4].

After this introduction a deep case history is taken using a schema devised by the director[5]. This is a four-page document which allows the patient to express their complaint in their own words as well as probing the effect upon their ailment of the time of day, weather conditions, social situations, heat, rest and foods. In addition it probes their 'mental or emotional make-up', as well as having the normal queries about the medical history of the patient and his or her family, and space for 'Physician's Notes' in which the results of medical tests can be written. After taking an hour to complete this case history the interviewer takes another hour to complete a 'repertory'. Using the schema the interviewer decides which are the ten most significant symptoms. Then, using these ten as a guide, he looks up the symptoms and their remedies in a book of homoeopathic medicine. Each remedy has a score of 1, 2 or 3. These scores are added together to arrive at the 'constitutional remedy'.

Finally active treatment starts - massage, relaxation, breathing exercises, physiotherapy, colonic irrigation, homoeopathic treatment and talk-to sessions centred around therapists. The (director) normally only comes down at weekends, his main practice is in London. The day-to-day work is done by therapists during the week...There are two girls, one of whom is a faith healer, a man who does acupuncture and psychotherapy, an osteopath and a radiesthesia laboratory...The spiritual element in it is undefined. Meditation ties in with breathing and relaxation. Homoeopathy tries to strengthen the whole person, get the body in tone - eating the right food is seen as part of it. Quite a bit is done by diet - nature cure - with fasting eliminating toxins...whole food is eaten...mainly vegan[4].

COLLEGE

A similar concern with digestion formed part of one treatment used by the director of the college of healing I visited:

(I) just had a girl suffering from a serious depression. I advised her to go and take a laxative and drink about four pints of dry cider, explaining the reasons for it. This (depression) is a sort of psycho-emotion produced by something I can't repeat but which happened last Sunday. And she now produced an engendering state of one organ affecting another and it's now affecting lungs and colon. For the psychological state of depression we feel nothing unless there's a physiological state which goes with it. That physiological state can be altered by stimulating lungs and by stimulating colon[6].

The prescription of laxative and dry cider for depression may not be standard medical practice but it was completely consistent with the healing theory of Michael Quentin-Hicks, the young director of the college. He explained to me that although he had a doctorate in psychology and had worked as a clinical psychotherapist he had decided that

the theory sounded nice...but it wasn't empirical enough, I couldn't see that it was obviously true...In the west we don't understand really. The mind and body are one thing...not two parts of one thing but completely one thing. Yin and Yang are two brains and the real brain is down there in the abdomen. The brain that calculates, that computes, doesn't produce any emotion, any feeling and it's emotion and feeling that makes human beings human. Also (it) is where they get into trouble too[6]. We don't have any patients who are psychological patients or any who are physical patients. Everybody's treated the same way as a person because they've all got the same disorder as far as we're concerned: they've got an imbalance of energies[7].

In line with his beliefs he had set up a trust:

The purpose of the trust is to run courses of natural healing therapies and bring such treatments to the public by opening new clinics wherever possible. This is also the college which runs courses varying in duration from four months to five years. These courses cover all aspects of natural medicine that can be used within the principles of oriental energic medicine; such as acupuncture, osteopathy, psycho-therapy, etc[8].

The college teaches by lecture and training sessions for those interested. A tape-recording of a lecture on examining the patient was kindly lent to me by the director and an edited version is given below:

First thing is to treat them with a certain amount of formality. They're nervous...and we need to reassure them...make them feel you are going to treat them with some form of confidence...Act out the part of being a consultant.

Always, at every time, speak with authority. Even if you don't know what the hell you're talking about it should always be said with an air of authority...If you're asked any questions you know the answer...Always got to be a positive answer...you should never say to anything you don't know.

Most of them are coming because they haven't had the right treatment elsewhere. Most people have been to GP's or been to hospital. They're still in pain...they must have, they're looking for that security of somebody who knows what's wrong with them and knows how to do it.

You can do that without being pompous...with this confidence...you're also going to attempt to be extremely gentle...without being sloppy about it...possibly adopting the role of a mother or father with a child...but of course a bit more polite than a mother or father would be to a child, but perhaps the same tone of voice, the same sort of attitude to them.

It's worth now studying and developing a professional personality, a professional manner, if you work in any clinic...it's going to be sixty per cent of the success of that place...

...You never laugh at a patient, you never do anything but agree with them whatever stupid thing they say. Also they are usually treated with such a great amount of detachment by other people, other places they've had treatment. They're treated so much as numbers...the fact that you're going to treat them entirely as an individual for half an hour, your undivided attention...if anything interrupts you, you apologize for that or you even put off the thing that's interrupting you.

Mr Zuckerman[9] comes...my accent becomes definitely yiddish. Couple of county people come, my accent becomes extremely county and I start to talk about yachting and horse-riding...if one of the county set comes in - you know, yacht club, country club, got their own boats, might have a couple of boats, sauna baths and that - you must immediately start talking on that level...If you can't afford horses, you can't afford power boats, it doesn't matter, you can always read books about them, can't you...you can know as much as you're supposed to know to hold a conversation about those things which are the everyday life of those people...adapting your own personality...that personality should be beyond social class, possessions or way of life.

...Be a reflection of the person you're treating...to be a more reliable, more secure part of themselves. So you're the rock, absolutely dependable, absolutely competent, absolutely sure of everything you do and as you're reflecting them they too can become sure of themselves.

....a white coat does give you the ability to change any way you like...because you are more or less detached from everyday life. Dress in reasonably clean attire to treat them as it's going to be seen as insulting (if you don't).

Examination is something which stops, starts...- according to what you're finding. Generally, leave pulses to fairly late on in the examination...(I get the) patient seated, put my hands on their shoulders, feeling the action of the shoulders, feeling the shoulders themselves.

On the first examination you must examine everything. During this time you can either chat or else look very serious and keep quiet.

While you're actually examining the back if you find anything particularly abnormal it's very reassuring to the patient if you say so...it's very important to them if you tell them what it is...they must be taken into the whole operation with you. Most of the people we see have a vague idea what's wrong with them. Unless I had a reasonable hope of success I wouldn't attempt to treat anything. People find this impressive and important.

Observe somebody's reaction to touch, observe their posture.

It impresses them that you're finding things without being told and this increases their confidence in you, which is important. Never take anybody else's opinion of what's wrong.

You can explain, if you know it, the process of what's going wrong with them...it's very reassuring and gives them a great deal of understanding and you get a great deal of co-operation in the treatment.

He explained the principle behind the mode of examination in this way:

If I say to somebody 'can you see the whole room?' they say 'yes', but if I'm talking to you, you look at me, (you) can't see the whole room. The only way to see the whole room is by not looking at anything. This is where the diagnosis is. We take pulses to find out how individual organs are working. We (are) probably examining skin colours, reflexes, gestures all at the same time...it's anything you can see about the person which is apparent. (You) ask what's wrong (but) not push it too far or they might clam up. At the same time form some opinion on the way they sit, the way they hold their hands, the way they use their eyes. Also listen to their words, (the) particular words they use...the basis of diagnosis really lies in the elements and the change of energy between organs...one emotion changes naturally to another[6].

I was also able to observe several training sessions. These took place in the clinic, a well-appointed set of rooms off a narrow alleyway near the centre of the city. The rooms have white walls and the floor is covered in green carpet. The main room in which the training session occurred, was about four yards wide by six yards long, and lit by two small windows of frosted glass. The furniture was scant: a single bed covered in a white sheet, a small bow table with a few bottles of surgical spirit and coconut oil on it between the windows, an armchair, two straight-backed chairs and a wardrobe in one corner. The bed had a fluorescent light over it. On the white walls were a large photograph of trees, a picture of a human body with Chinese

characters written all over it and a framed picture of a
male nude.

In the room there were six people (apart from myself):
Michael, the director, standing at the foot of the bed,
Christopher[10], a tall well-built man in his early forties,
sitting on the bed, Joan and Carole at the side of the bed
sitting on the floor with their backs to the wall (Joan was
about twenty years old, Carole was probably about thirty),
Rebecca standing next to them (also about thirty years old),
and finally, set apart from the others, Doris, who was
sitting on a hard-backed chair next to the wardrobe (she was
blind and in her late forties). As I settled down to take
notes they were all discussing the symptoms that someone had
presented.

REBECCA: I've got a splitting head. Michael can you massage
    my head?
CAROLE: Your headache's coming from your neck.
MICHAEL: Can you make some tea, Carole? What are we going to
    do?
CHRISTOPHER: What happened to Lucy? She had acupuncture and
    massage.
MICHAEL: She was quite fit yesterday., I warn my patients we
    don't have any treatments which just take the symptoms
    off.
CHRISTOPHER: (sceptically): What's macro-biotics?
MICHAEL: It's balancing elements.
CHRISTOPHER: Varied diet, set of pulses a lot stronger.
MICHAEL: (to all): 'Anything unusual?'
DORIS: Pains in my arm.
MICHAEL: Doris first. (Doris comes over and sits on the bed
    with help from the others.) Look at Doris's arms first.
    (Michael is probing in the back of Doris's neck and the
    others are crowding around to look.) Damp weather - it's
    muscular rheumatism.
    (Christopher volunteers to diagnose and treat. Michael
    continues by taking pulses.) It's a spinal problem but
    generally better than you had. (Carole comes in with the
    tea which is without milk or sugar. Michael continues to
    treat Doris. He keeps hold of her with one hand while
    moving around with the other. He starts to discuss a
    previous case which has come to mind during his
    observation of Doris.) She was a young woman coming in
    with arthritis. STM - soft tissue manipulation - was
    effective.

Doris lies face down on the bed and takes off her top and
bra. Christopher gets coconut oil on his hands and squeezes
her back. As he does this Carole makes an appointment to
bring in her four year-old youngster, Michael says, 'Kids
are very easy to treat. They get better much quicker than
grown-ups.' Christopher asks if he's rubbing away the
fibrous mass and Michael says, 'It won't get rid of it all.
Doris probably, like most of us, needs regular treatment.'

Michael meanwhile is massaging Joan's back as she stands

watching. She blushes. Doris sits up and Michael moves her backwards and forwards, getting her to twist her body. When she lies down again Christopher again massages her back.

At this point Jack arrives. He, like Christopher, is in his early forties. Carole goes off to make some more tea and Doris gets up and dresses.

Michael calls Joan to come and sit on the bed. She's shy and sits rather rigidly. She tells them she's not been sleeping well. As she does so Rebecca holds one hand, Michael the other, but he's called away to see a patient so Christopher holds her hand. She begins to relax as Michael returns and tells her she's physically overactive.

'Reflexes', says Michael and she takes all the clothing off the top of her body and lies down on the bed on her back. Michael massages her lower abdomen while they all look on, asking how to tell what's wrong. Michael says, 'Nothing wrong with Joan. Thing's are going right, you're just adjusting.'

Jack asks if he can have a go, Michael replies jokingly, 'I'll do it, with pleasure, too. I can't keep my hands off Joan.' Jack starts to massage after Joan has turned on her stomach. During all this Christopher is the only one taking notes.

Carole tells Joan, 'I believe your back is a better shape Joan, since you first came.' Michael recommends a homoeopathic medicine and tells Joan where to get it. Rebecca takes over the massage from Jack. There is a phone call for Jack, and Christopher is talking to Doris. Rebecca starts to clean the oil from Joan's back with surgical spirit.

Jack volunteers to be the guinea pig and takes off his shirt and vest. Michael holds one hand and Joan the other. Carole and Rebecca look on. Michael tells me, 'We're not a bunch of hypochondriacs, we just practise on each other on Tuesday afternoons.'

Doris is brought over to take pulses. David, lying on his back, complains of just being 'generally out of sorts'. Michael tells them all that 'pulse and reflexes are the most important, you can't look at them too often.' Rebecca starts massaging while Carole looks on. While this is taking place Joan is explaining yin/yang pulses to Christopher.

Michael says he's going to use needles. The massage is hurting Jack as it goes on.

When I asked him why he was going to use needles then, he replied that the 'body electricities need a lot more investigation'. Michael then takes several small needles and pushes them into Jack. Jack tells them all 'the whole thing was released right round the front. It felt like a sort of wave, a release of tension.'

After the needles are removed there is some banter between Carole and Christopher over who is to continue the massage, Carole starts to prepare but Christopher says, 'I'll do it,' to which Carole replies, 'I'll pinch the oil. I've never had a go at him before.' Christopher says he wants to compare how he is now from when he treated him last week. Eventually Joan massages with Carole advising her — 'Can you feel the fibre?' — and then Rebecca. Finally Christopher takes a turn.

Michael tells me he used to work with another acupuncturist but left the partnership five years ago because the partner 'became so involved with money. We charge enough to provide a reasonable living. We are only the instrument, we perform something that already exists. Once you start thinking you're very good at this that's the end.'

BALANCE AND HARMONY

The explanations which see healing as the restoration of harmony in the individual, homoeopathy, and such notions as yin and yang, are sophisticated intellectual elaborations of the folk beliefs of peasant societies. Such beliefs are often seen as 'eastern' beliefs and, by those that hold them, much is made of their long history in Chinese and Indian thought. However, such beliefs are not confined to the East. They were a normal part of western society when it was predominantly a peasant society (see Thomas, 1973) and they remain part of the beliefs of peasant societies in the West today. Thus in Mexico (see Ingham, 1970) folk medicine sees the balancing of 'hot' and 'cold' as vital for good health. 'Hot' and 'cold' are attributes, not only of the temperature but of food and feeling. The concept does not refer to the heat foods gain from cooking but to a quality integral to them (e.g. some herbs are hot and some are cold regardless of how they are cooked). Similarly 'hot' passions have nothing to do with body temperature. Envy, malice and sexual excitement are all seen as 'hot' passions which can cause damage. Illness is seen as a result of an imbalance in a person's moral or social state and the cure is sought in restoration of harmony[11]. Such beliefs are integrally bound up with the peasant's way of life and his conception of that life as a 'zero sum game'. That is, he believes that in this world there are only so many good things available — so much land, so much rain, so much sun, so much happiness, so much honour, so much health — and so if one person gets more of the fixed cake of happiness, someone else is sure to get less. This image of the limited good[12] means that a peasant wishing to live a good moral life must continually seek a balance between fulfilling his own desires and harming his neighbour. If he were to gain too much — too much land, too much money, too much luck, too much good health — then his neighbour, according to his belief, would

98

have less. The idea of balance pervades all aspects of peasant belief, including health and illness. A man who has good health attributes it to the grace of God, a gift, and he attributes ill-health to his failure to maintain a balanced, moderate life. Alternatively, he may attribute his ill-health to the jealousy of neighbours - the witchcraft we have already encountered in the Philippines and which is such a pervasive feature in one form or another in peasant societies[13]. The treatment in either case is to seek to capture or recapture harmony. Harmony within the individual, harmony within the community, and harmony within the cosmos. For it must be emphasised that in peasant societies the line between the individual, the community and the cosmos is not as sharply drawn as it is in industrial society. In the words of the Blums (1965) discussing Greek peasants:

> The child has learned to strongly identify with the lives of others in his family. Reared as he has been and will be, in such a manner that being with and part of others is his only experience, he has little 'private self' that allows him to objectify what is physically and emotionally his versus what is another's. The difference between mother and child, which Americans prize as a developmental goal, is not a Greek concern. The personality, the self of the child, is formed not just by associating with others but by merging with them. Consequently, a person is produced who not only is family oriented, highly sociable, and internally supported in crises by indivisible affiliations with others but is also highly vulnerable to the ills, moods and evils of others; for him being alone is loneliness, and loneliness is terror, for without the company of others he feels that part of himself is gone.

In fact to talk of an individual separate from his social context is ludicrous in such a society and medical practices which try to treat individuals in this manner are fundamentally at variance with the people they seek to help[14]. Treatment is the restoration of harmony within the individual and thus within his social group.

It is from such societies and such ideals that the 'eastern' beliefs and practices described in this chapter originated. That is not to dismiss them as peasant or folk beliefs for such beliefs are becoming increasingly popular in the 'West'. They owe their acceptance in the 'West' to a shift in some aspects of western belief which have occurred since the Second World War, especially in the USA. This shift was discussed and elaborated by David Riesman et al. (1950) when they distinguished a move in the USA from a society in which individuals were expected to be guided by their individual consciences, 'inner-directed' men, to a society where individuals are guided by their fellows, 'other-directed' men. In Britain the popularity of Laing's work on schizophrenia (Laing, 1972) (which suggests that it is a social not an individual condition, that the schizophrenic is acting rationally in response to an intolerable social situation) signals a similar shift towards looking at the social context of individuals, rather than their internal states, to explain their actions and I shall, in fact, be adopting a similar sociological framework to explain healing in the final chapter of the book. However, before doing that we need to look at further explanations of healing - both those put forward by healers and those put forward by orthodox medicine and this constitutes the next chapter.

NOTES

(1) The name Ramana refers to the Director's own philosophical/religious beliefs, which entail an enquiry into the self. While I was at the hospital I observed a religious service to Rama (in the library/chapel) during which the question 'Who am I?' was reiterated many times. It is the belief of the Director that the continuous question 'Who am I?' produces peace in those hearing it. The library/chapel is used also for other religious services, by other faiths, and contains a curved apse (on which a madonna is mounted ouside the building) and an altar which has a cross and a buddha on it.
(2) From a pamphlet of the centre.
(3) From an interview with the director.
(4) Interview with a nurse. This was not tape-recorded so is not verbatim.
(5) A copy was given to me by the director's personal assistant.
(6) Interview with the director.
(7) From a lecture on energic anatomy - a tape of the lecture was kindly lent by the director.
(8) From the centre's prospectus.
(9) Pseudonym.
(10) A pseudonym as are the other names.
     Christopher is a 52 year-old insurance salesman married with one child. He came originally because of a back injury. He was passing and noticed the sign, osteopath. He now wants to help others with back problems.
     Joan is a young woman who'd left university and was unemployed. Carole is 32, married to a self-employed carpenter and has two children. She came as a student. Rebecca is a young woman. Doris is blind, single and in her forties. Jack is a headmaster for a junior school, aged 39 with three children. He came for treatment and its effect was dramatic and beneficial so he decided to follow it up.
(11) See Blum and Blum (1965). Also see Fabrega (1970) and Colson (1976) for accounts of the notion of balance in peasant societies.
(12) Foster (1965) uses this phrase in the article which first set out this idea in detail.
(13) Another variant is the 'evil eye'. See Blum and Blum (1965) and Ingham (1970).
(14) Manning and Fabrega (1973) give an extensive account of this clash.

6 How does healing work?

At the end of the first chapter I concluded by saying that
the question 'How does healing work?' would have to be held
in abeyance until we had examined many more healers than the
Filipino psychic surgeons. We have now almost reached the
end of the healing therapies and theories that will be
described in this book. These descriptions are inadequate
reflections of the richness of real experiences, and
although not all the healing therapies I observed are
described (indeed, they are but a fraction of the total
healing therapies available), nonetheless .they provide
sufficient information to enable us to return to the
question - how does healing work?

The healers we have looked at provide three types of
explanation. They explain healing (a) as the result of
supernatural intervention, (b) as the result of natural
forces or (c) as the restoration of harmony in the afflicted
individual. We have already looked in some detail, in the
preceding chapter, at the idea that healing is the
restoration of harmony so there is no need to retrace our
steps in that particular terrain. However, it is important
to realise there is no clear dividing line between these
three types of explanation: those who believe in
supernatural intervention usually qualify their belief by
asserting that although the intervention is supernatural the
means used by the supernatural being are natural; those who
talk of natural forces also talk of a spiritual world; and
those who talk of supernatural beings also stress wholeness
and balance.

Let us look first at supernatural intervention. The
fundamental feature of supernatural healing is that the
healing is seen to come from outside. The healing 'power' is
a gift of God or spirits which is granted to an individual
or a place. The individual who has the gift does not seek
it. The individual healer or the place of healing are
'channels' through which the healing power flows. They are
normally seen to have no power in themselves[1]. This
description of healing as a result of supernatural
intervention is a gross over-simplification however.
Although all healers who account for healings as a

consequence of supernatural intervention appear to do so in these terms, they also have a variety of other themes, which will be taken up later when giving a sociological explanation. In particular they often stress that cure is a function of the Church acting as a community, e.g., Wilson (1966) argues that 'The unit of the Church's healing is the local congregation' and 'such an accepting family life, in home or church or community has the power to heal', while Lambourne (1963) argues that the Church should be a therapeutic community. Similarly McNutt gives an extensive quotation describing 'miracle services' in which

> a community of love and acceptance is created. People feel secure enough to lay aside the barriers of fear, distrust and egotism that have shut them off not only from fruitful contact with their fellow men but from their own deeper selves. There is a yielding up of self-isolation. The individual loses himself in the group, the symbol of the loving family where one is accepted in spite of his faults and sins. He identifies with the needs of others. He sometimes forgets his own illness, his own needs, in praying for someone else whose need is greater. in this self-forgetfulness, as it happens, he is healed.' (McNutt, 1974, quoting Spraggett, 1970).

This quotation raises another theme that runs through supernatural explanations, that of the individual as linked with others and as changing because of healing. Wilson expresses this theme when he says 'we belong to one another; there is no such thing as a separate person', and 'sickness is a learning situation...none of them (patient, doctor, family) emerges from the situation as the same person'. (Wilson, 1966) These notions of the healing being accomplished by the church acting as a community and the transformation of the individual remain, however, sub-themes in the supernatural explanation of healing. They are as it were 'working theories' of what actually takes place rather than metatheories of the mechanism of healing. This remains as a gift of God or the action of supernatural beings, although as Harry Edwards points out such beings act through natural forces:

> When a physical change takes place...the result follows the application of law-governed energies or forces to make the chemical change. To operate that there must be an intelligence that has the ability of diagnosing one. Secondly it must have the ability of getting those energies together in their right strength...and as that intelligence is not human, because no human mind has this ability, that does prove in my mind the existence of another realm of intelligence, which we call the spirit world. (See Chapter 2)

Although spiritual and religious healers see healing as the action of natural forces, they see them as operated by supernatural forces. There are other healers, however, who would argue that there is no need to posit a supernatural realm. They see healing as the operation of natural forces of which we have only an imperfect understanding. The clearest exponents of this view are those practising radionics. Such people usually seek to measure this natural force and attempts to measure it provide Maxwell Cade with a fruitful field of study. Maxwell Cade has had an interesting and productive life. He was a zen student before going up to Guy's hospital as a medical student. His studies at Guy's were interrupted by the Second World War and he became involved in the development of radar for the RAF. After the war he went into the civilian application of radar, entered the Navy briefly, returned to civilian life, joining a firm which was eventually taken over by Smiths, the major British instrument makers. In time he became their chief medical physicist and a Fellow of the Royal Society of Medicine, Member of the Institute of Biology, Member of the Institute of Physics and a Fellow of the Institution of Electrical Engineers[2]. This job came to an abrupt end when he became blind. He was, however, healed and now concentrates some of his considerable talents on studying healing[3]. He does this by utilising a device which he and Geoff Blundell developed with the aid of a grant from the Healing Research Trust[4]. The instrument they developed is a box, called a 'Mind Mirror', which looks something like an elaborate control mechanism for a hi-fi unit. Within the box are controls and a display panel. The display panel consists of twelve rows of small lights which are connected via electrodes to the left side of the brain and a parallel set of twelve which are connected to the right hand side of the brain. The rows light up according to brain-wave activity: in ascending order they show delta waves, theta waves, alpha waves and beta waves[5]. The Mind Mirror is a sophisticated electroencephalograph which gives a read-out by patterns of flashing lights rather than the more conventional read-out on graph paper utilising a pen and a revolving drum. The advantage claimed for the Mind Mirror over the conventional e.e.g. machine is that the analysis of a conventional e.e.g. graph is so complex that a person cannot be asked his subjective feelings at the time the graph is being produced. The Mind Mirror by contrast displays a pattern of brain-waves as they are produced and so a direct link can be made with subjective feelings. The patterns produced can be interpreted:

Table 3

The Stages of Awareness[6]

Stage	Name	Description	Mind mirror patterns
0	Deep sleep		
1	Dreaming sleep		
2	Hypnagogic state	Between waking and sleeping: reverie	
3	Waking; waking sleep (Gurdjieff)	Ordinary awareness	
4	Fourth state (Wallace); meditation (traditional)	Very calm detached awareness, both internal and external	
5	Fifth state (Goleman); after glow (Mahirishi); illumination (Fromm); lucid awareness (Cade)	Great alertness yet calmly detached. Voluntary control of internal states (e.g. pain) greatly enhanced.	
6	Creativity	Great control, both internal and external. Sometimes spontaneous reduction or disappearance of physical symptoms of disease or injury	
7	Psychedelic (Gowan); illumination (Bucke); self-remembering (Gurdjieff)	Transcendence? (descriptions of this state are given on pp.132-134)	?
8	Cosmic consciousness	Transcendence?	?

104

Cade and his co-workers claim that the fifth state is characteristic of healers when treating their patients and that patients adopt this pattern of brain-waves when being treated. They also argue that healers can, by the use of the Mind Mirror, improve their effectiveness by seeing if their actions are producing changes in brain-wave patterns in their patients and modifying their actions accordingly. I was able to observe him using this device at a healing session run by Major Macmanaway in an 'artisan's cottage' in London. 'Artisan's cottage' is the term estate agents use for what was in fact a workman's terraced house in London. Today they are beyond the pocket of any workman, nor would the original occupants recognise it as the same house: what was the paved backyard has been converted into a walled garden with potted plants everywhere, and what was the cellar in which the milk was kept cool and coal stored has become a carpeted basement. He might perhaps recognise the old kitchen table which has been stripped down to the bare wood, as have all the doors, but apart from those remnants of the old house all would be strange. The change in the house echoes the change in the residents. Both the healer and his clients move in a world where the client asks that his next consultation be re-arranged so that he can go to Ascot Week and requests advice on which boarding school to send a child to.

Bruce Macmanaway, the main healer, was a tall well-built man who dominated the gathering. As an officer at Dunkirk he found

> he had the power to remove pain and staunch the flow
> of blood from serious wounds. Before his retirement
> from the army he had a bad motor cycling accident
> which, according to medical opinion, should have left
> him partially blind and crippled. Through healing by
> Harry Edwards and the White Eagle Lodge he made an
> astonishing and complete recovery. He has been a
> full-time healer since 1959...practising healing,
> special connection, nerve release, deep muscle
> therapy, meditation, dowsing, development of E.S.P.
> faculty, food reform and relaxation[7].

Maxwell Cade is a shorter, stockier individual. Whereas Bruce Macmanaway gave the impression of striding from place to place, Maxwell Cade glided there. Both, once they got where they were going, were still and calm.

The healing session was largely conducted in the drawing room, sited in the front of the house at street level. It had windows front and rear and was well lit by natural light. By the rear window there was a small area occupied by a bureau that formed a kind of office. The centre of the room was a collection of upholstered furniture grouped around an unlit fireplace. As well as Bruce Macmanaway and Maxwell Cade there were a number of other helpers present. Helping Maxwell Cade were his wife Isabel and Geoff Blundell, the technician who developed the Mind Mirror with

Maxwell Cade. Geoff and Isabel did most of the connecting up
of the machine to people, using small contacts that attached
to the skull, and they were often engaged in a flurry of
activity. They were not mere technical assistants, however,
and they too acted as healers sometimes. Both were warm
personalities and contrast with Bruce Macmanaway and Maxwell
Cade who remained somewhat distant in their interactions.
There were others also present at various times - a
newspaper reporter in his late twenties or early thirties
who initially came on assignment and kept coming out of
interest, two well-dressed slim women in early middle age,
Archie, another healer, and of course the patients.

One patient I observed being treated by the laying on of
hands and radiesthesia was Malcolm[8], a child of about nine
years old. He was connected to a Mind Mirror by Isabel and
Bruce Macmanaway was connected to another Mind Mirror:

B. MACMANAWAY: Hello (to father). Hello, Malcolm have
    a good Easter?
FATHER: Bruce, he's still not hearing very well.
B. MACMANAWAY: He was.
FATHER: He was, it comes and goes. Noticed latterly he's
    not been hearing well at particular angles.
(Geoff tries some rough testing of the child's hearing
    by snapping his fingers and Isabel persuades Malcolm
    to sit in a chair that is lower and more comfortable
    for his size.)
M. CADE (to me): I'm seeing if Bruce is tired by checking
    his brain waves.
B. MACMANAWAY (TO M. CADE): You say, if you want extra
    people brought in.
(Bruce has his hands either sides of Malcolm's ears but
    doesn't touch the ears. Max and Geoff are both
    watching the machine intently.)
FATHER: Oh, Max, he's cut down on the drug, one spoonful
    only.
(Bruce is now touching Malcolm and looking to see if the
    pattern on the Mind Mirror changes (it doesn't).
    Geoff puts a hand on Bruce's shoulder.)
FATHER (to me): Improvement has been dramatic since
    treatment started last December.
(Isabel is now touching Geoff. Bruce takes his hands off
    and crosses them. Behind me three women are talking
    quietly, otherwise everyone is silent. Malcolm
    has now closed his eyes.)
ISABEL: He's improving here.
(Max goes round and places one hand on Geoff and one on
    Bruce. There is thus a whole train of people. Geoff
    asks for the contacts to be moved on Bruce. Apparently
    the reporter who wired Bruce up did them back to front.
    Isabel does it and she and Geoff whisper about it.
    One of the other women comes along and adds yet
    another person to 'the train' by putting her hand on
    Geoff's shoulder.

All this time the father has been standing by the
fireplace.
    Geoff moves one hand until it is over the hand of
Bruce and then he moves it about.
    The child has now been sitting still for fifteen
minutes. Bruce moves his hand over the child's chest,
rests there for a while, then moves underneath the
child's arm coming back to rest on the abdomen.
    Max sits down to look at the Mind Mirror.
    The father opens his diary.
    Both Bruce and Geoff have their eyes closed. The
woman removes her hands, rubs them together, then
returns them to Geoff's shoulders; closing her eyes
again.
    Malcolm is now fidgeting, obviously getting bored.
Bruce moves his hands again until they are crossed
across the back of Malcolm's neck and are resting on
his shoulders.
    Isabel is talking quietly to Max about the display
on the Mind Mirror. Apart from these two the child
is the centre of attention in a silent room.
    Bruce massages Malcolm's shoulders and his father
moves round to look over Max's shoulder at the
display.
    There is an interruption to the silence when Archie
(another healer) emerges with a client from another
room and sees him to the front door.
    Bruce moves his hands back to the position he
started from, either side of the head, but not
touching and then touches the top of the head.
    The father is talking to Max and says hello to
Archie.
    Bruce now opens his eyes and talks to the father
in whispers. Isabel chats to the woman who joined
'the train' of healers.
    The father goes back to the fireplace and looks
at Malcolm.)
B. MACMANAWAY: Max, did any one point of contact produce
    more effect?
(Geoff steps away.
    Bruce moves his hands, front and back of Malcolm.)
ISABEL: There is a response wherever you touch but
    there were longer Delta today. (i.e. Delta waves
    were sustained for a long period)
B. MACMANAWAY: One hopes.
GEOFF (To Bruce): You seem to be better.
ISABEL: More Delta flares from Bruce today.
(Bruce is now using keys as a pendulum on the child's
back.
    Two more patients arrive and are asked to go down
    to the basement. They know the father of Malcolm and
    say hello.
    Bruce now leans back from Malcolm.
    Malcolm is still hooked up and is smiling.)
ISABEL: With Malcolm's eyes closed he's going into the
    fifth state.
B. MACMANAWAY: Max, can you explain the fifth state to

107

Malcolm's father. With luck I may talk myself out
of a job.
(Bruce, Max and the father go toward the office part of
the room. The father is asking Bruce for advice
about Malcolm going to boarding school, Bruce says
that it is fine. He takes a cheque for 12 pounds
from the father who says, 'It is cheap at the
price'.)
MAX (to father): He's started to produce patterns
himself.
FATHER: He's catching up?
MAX: He's beginning to get himself straight...(and he
goes on to explain the fifth state).
FATHER: Things are going wonderful well.
(While the dialogue was going on in 'the office' one
woman put her hands on Malcolm's shoulders and
another woman held his clasped hands.)
WOMAN 1 (to Geoff): Is this the way to do it?
GEOFF: Yes, if you're getting any feeling.
WOMAN 2 (to Malcolm): How old are you, are you nine?
MALCOLM: Yes.
(Isabel now joins them and asks Malcolm to do some
reading for her. The father is now reading a
journal and is not looking at the child any more.
Isabel is getting Malcolm to remember things,
particularly colours. Malcolm looks to his father
for approval of his success but his father is not
looking. The father, the reporter and myself are the
only men left in the room by now.)
WOMAN 2: Has it changed?
ISABEL (for Malcolm): It's strengthening, it's
strengthening the whole time.
FATHER (to woman): By the time he comes again he'll be
cut down on dose. He's been on the drug for five
or six years. Since January the improvement has
been tremendous.
WOMAN 1 (for Malcolm): Isn't it lovely to have someone
so responsive.
FATHER (to woman): Lots of our friends noticed.
WOMAN 2 (for Malcolm): It shows credit to Malcolm. He's
always terribly patient.
(Malcolm is looking down at the display on the Mind
Mirror which since Max left the room has been on
the floor in front of him.)
ISABEL: Do you feel tickles and prickles?
MALCOLM: No.
ISABEL: Is it pleasant?
(Malcolm nods his head in agreement.)
WOMAN 2 (holding hands splayed behind child): Had enough?
(Malcolm nods.)
WOMAN 2 (Gets him to sit up straighter. He's gradually
been slumping in the chair): Can you feel nice and
balanced? You're sitting crooked. I think he's had
enough.
FATHER: Try and sit up straight!
(At this point I left the room to observe elsewhere.)

Through using the Mind Mirror Cade has demonstrated to his own satisfaction and to others that a change in a healer produces a change in a patient; the patient's pattern of brain waves gradually synchronizes with those of the healer when the healer lays hands upon the patient. In North America also there is evidence that the healer produces change[9]. This evidence has been produced by a series of controlled experiments. It started with a set of experiments undertaken by a laboratory technician in Montreal, Bernie Grad[10]. He inflicted wounds of a standard size on mice by removing a portion of their skin. He then had a healer lay hands upon half the mice individually. This was done by having the mice in individual cages covered in a paper bag. The mice to be 'treated' were chosen randomly and neither the experimenter nor the healer knew which mice were to be used, nor until the experiment was completed did they know which mice had been chosen. This technique, known technically as a double-blind experiment in that both the experimenter and the subject are 'blind', ensures as far as is possible that bias towards a result on the part of subject or experimenter can be avoided. After a period of time the size of the wound on each mouse was measured and then the group which had been 'treated' was compared with the other group, the control group, which had not been treated. The mice that had been 'treated' had significantly[11] smaller wounds when compared with the untreated mice.

Later experiments produced a better plant yield from plants watered with water that had been held in the hand of a healer. This research was extended by Sister M. Justa Smith, who demonstrated changes in the enzyme trypsin after it had been treated by the same healer[12], and by Dolores Krieger, a nurse, who obtained statistically significant results when the same healer held flasks containing haemaglobin (Krieger, 1975). Krieger, in an extension of this experiment, had a control and experimental group of nurses (sixteen in each group) in which the experimental group practised laying-on-of-hands; this experiment also produced a statistically significant change in haemaglobin. One might well ask, given these results, why laying on of hands is not widely accepted as a therapeutic technique by orthodox doctors. I think the answer lies in the fact that it does not fit into the prevailing medical or scientific paradigm. Science operates not in terms of an individual proceeding with an open mind but in terms of individuals operating within a set of rules which decide which are the problems worth considering and how they are to be tackled. Polanyi, a scientist and philosopher of science, expresses the point well:

There must be at all times a predominantly accepted scientific view of the nature of things, in the light of which research is jointly conducted by members of the community of scientists. A strong presumption that any evidence which contradicts this view is invalid must prevail. Such evidence has to be

109

disregarded, even if it cannot be accounted for, in the hope that it will eventually turn out to be false or irrelevant[13].

However, orthodox medicine, like science, is generally not favourable to any of these explanations of how 'alternative' healing works - whether they be supernatural forces, forces unknown to science, or the need to restore harmony. In fact when faced with such explanations the response of orthodox medicine is to dismiss cures produced by alternative practices as spontaneous remission, to see them as a consequence of a placebo effect or to see such cures as produced by a primitive form of psychotherapy.

Spontaneous remission is not so much an explanation as an admission that doctors are unable to provide an explanation. To call an unexpected cure a spontaneous remission is merely to relabel it, not to explain it. Consequently those doctors who do report such cases (e.g. Kessell, 1959) comment on the paucity of the literature and admit they cannot explain their findings.

The literature on the placebo effect is much more interesting. The word placebo is usually taken to mean a 'sugar pill' (in fact it is Latin for 'I will please') but the literature on the topic uses the term in a much wider sense to mean any therapeutic practice which has no clear clinical effect. The systematic medical interest in placebos started in the 1950s (see Wolf, 1950; Wolf and Pinsky, 1954; Lasagna et al., 1954; and Beecher, 1955). Research workers found that inert medications were able to relieve pain in approximately one-third of their sample suffering from a variety of illnesses ranging from post-operative pain to the common cold. In 1956 two researchers, Fisher and Olin, reported a study in which they compared three groups of mentally ill patients who were treated by a placebo, a 'mind drug' and by psychotherapy. The most successful treatment was psychotherapy, which produced improvement in 61 per cent of the patients. However, 47 per cent of the mind drug group and 42 per cent of the patients given a placebo also improved. To explain the operation of the placebo, they argued that it was not just the inert medication, the placebo, that produced the improvement in the patients but the doctor-patient relationship: 'all humans...may as a result of suffering and longing for relief, obtain a placebo reaction to the medication regardless of its nature. Especially may the response include varying amounts of placebo reaction if the healer is held in great esteem.'

By 1964, Shapiro, in a summary article, was able to cite clear evidence that placebos could affect organic illnesses, including malignancies that were presumed to be incurable[14]. Reviewing the experimental and clinical literature he argued that the key factor in the placebo response appeared to be the doctor-patient relationship. When the patient trusted the doctor, and when the doctor believed in the treatment he was employing and was interested, confident, friendly, reassuring and thorough, then the placebo reaction appeared. There appeared to be little or no relationship to patient variables and the suggestibility of the patient was not related to the effect. However, the more impressive the treatment method, the more likely the placebo response. What Shapiro's article implies is that the placebo reaction is one produced by a social context rather than the result of personality variation. However, more recent work, summarised by Jospe (1978, pp.90,147), forces a modification of this picture by distinguishing studies that used patients from studies that used non-patients. It appears, when this is done, that patients who react to placebos do have certain characteristics:

> they are people who depend upon, and trust in, other
> people's ability to help them. In view of their
> religiousness, the belief that others can help them
> does not extend only to mortals...The placebo
> reactors place much reliance on others to be the
> agents in their therapeutic change. They are anxious,
> field dependent, talkative, and emotionally labile.
> They cannot get along well with other people, even
> though at times they allow themselves to be dominated
> by others, especially authority figures

Nonetheless it is not a sufficient explanation of the placebo response to dismiss it as an effect produced only in suggestible individuals. The placebo effect is 'a product of the interaction between patient-personality-placebo-healer-situation variables' as Jospe puts it.

The clearest use of the placebo interpretation of alternative medicine is contained in Katz's (1972) attack upon chiropractic where he dismisses it as a placebo, contrasting it with conventional medicine which, he argues, does not rely on the placebo effect. Works such as those described by Jospe and the type of work undertaken by Comaroff (1976) who demonstrated that the use of pills in general practice has many of the characteristics of placebo therapy in that it reassures patient <u>and</u> doctor that something is being done, suggests that the distinction drawn by Katz between orthodox and alternative medicine is not as clear in practice as it is in theory. All therapists appear to be enjoying a placebo effect whether they are orthodox, alternative or traditional.

The interpretation of 'faith-healing' as a form of 'primitive' psychotherapy has formed the major medical explanation of healing[15]. This literature normally distinguishes psychotherapy from faith-healing in terms of the aims of the therapy; psychotherapy is seen as seeking insight and independence on the part of the patient whereas faith healing seeks belief and dependence (see, e.g. Prince, 1972). Not all those practising alternative medicine would agree, however. For example a former doctor at Burrswood stressed the independence healing gives compared with psychotherapy:

The psychiatrist says in effect to his patient: this
is why you are as you are, you are not to blame. This
may be true, and it may be right for the patient (and
those who suffer from his bad behaviour) to know it.
But this knowledge often leads no further than
despair, self-pity or evasion of reality. Something
more is needed. The patient must be convinced that he
need not be limited by his past, that it will not
help to excuse his behaviour on the basis of
impulses, habits and unconscious motives of which he
is the helpless victim. He must be helped to become
responsible. He must be made to face the issue of
right and wrong. He must stop looking backwards: he
must turn round: he must be 'converted'. He must have
a goal towards which he can strive with heart, mind
and will[16].

Similarly Calestro (1972) makes no such distinction and sees
both faith-healing and psychotherapy as involved in
'secondary suggestibility', i.e. 'change in an individual's
cognitive or perceptual behaviour (or both) as a result of
subjective interpersonal influence'. Such a change is
produced when both healer and patient share the same
presumptions about the world, when the healer is granted
high expertise and credibility by the patient, and he is
seen as sincere and trustworthy. Although there is some
evidence of individual differences in suggestibility, it
appears that 'situational factors involving the identity of
the individual making the suggestion, the context of the
suggestion and the personal involvement of the audience
appear to be vital factors.' One situational factor stands
out as important in all the work on psychotherapy and that
is that the process includes a period of 'chaos' when the
patient is unsure of himself: 'an individual's
susceptibility to interpersonal influence...is increased
when he finds himself in an unfamiliar or ambiguous
situation.'

CONCLUSION

Both the medical work on placebos and the medical analysis
of healing as a form of psychotherapy suggest a similar
mechanism is in operation when healing takes place. That
mechanism is a function of the social context and in
particular of the healer-patient relationship. Social
context and social relationships are also seen as important
by the healers themselves, regardless of whether they are
Christian, spiritualist, 'Eastern' or radiesthetic healers.
This is not to imply that they see social relationships as
paramount. Their theories variously stress spirits, Christ,
magnetic forces and balancing yin and yang, and in this they
differ profoundly from each other. However, their working
theories, that is their comments on how they actually set
about healing people and their actions in doing such
healing, are remarkably similar. They all concern themselves

with social relationships. Given this fact it seems more than time that sociological explanations of healing were examined and such explanations will form the theme of the next and final chapter.

NOTES

(1) This idea has been expressed in one form or another by all the spiritualist and Christian healers in this book.
(2) This information was given in interview and in the back of Cade and Coxhead (1979).
(3) He is primarily interested in bio-feedback.
(4) The Healing Research Trust is an organisation of individuals interested in promoting and researching into alternative medicine.
(5) A picture of the instrument appears on p. 9 of Cade and Coxhead (1979).
(6) Adapted from EEG Measurement published by Audio Ltd. 26 Wendell Road, London, by kind permission.
(7) Taken from the programme notes of the sixth annual conference of the Wrekin Trust on 'Health and Healing'.
(8) A pseudonym.
(9) There is other evidence from the USA that the healer changes during healing. A group of researchers, led by Dr Thelma Moss, in California, have been trying to take 'photographs' of the 'energy' of healers. To accomplish this they use a technique called Kirlian photography which demonstrates a different colour and strength of rays emitted from a healer's hands before, during and after a healing session. Accounts of this work are contained in the publication of the Academy of Parapsychology and Medicine (1972); an extensive bibliography on the subject can be obtained from Dr Moss at UCLA and a picture taken by Kirlian photography can be seen in Kingston (1975).
(10) See Grad (1961 and 1967); Krieger (1975).
(11) As measured by standard statistical tests.
(12) Smith (1972). She was not able to replicate this however - see Eagle (1978).
(13) Cited in Stent (1978). See Kuhn (1962) for a discussion of scientific paradigms and Stent (1978) for a discussion of the way in which evidence is not enough to ensure scientific acceptance of a phenomena; the phenomena has to fit into the prevailing paradigm or await the construction of a new paradigm into which it does fit.
(14) Shapiro (1964). In fact one of the earliest studies of placebo reaction - Wolf (1950) - had demonstrated that placebos have a physiological effect.
(15) The most prominent exponents of this view are Ari Kiev (1964, 1966a, 1966b). William Sargant (1959) and, especially, Frank (1963) although it underlies many other interpretations of group healing rituals in which the trance states of patients are interpreted as abreaction e.g. Holland and Tharp (1964).
(16) From 'Where Religion and Science Meet', undated pamphlet written by Dr E.A. Aubert MD of Burrswood.

7 What is Man?

Sociological studies of healing have so far looked at affliction as - and only as - a social event. They have left the study of the organic changes involved to doctors and the psychological changes to psychologists and psychiatrists. Their concern has been with the different things different societies call 'sickness'. (See Eisenberg, 1977; Frankenberg and Leeson, 1976; Kleinman, 1973, Kleinman and Sung, 1976, Lewis, 1975.) They have been interested in the social variation in the criteria used for recognising affliction. Those criteria are:

(1) objective damage as recognised using special instruments or procedures;
(2) manifest signs of impaired functioning;
(3) the patient's feeling of unease (Lewis, 1953).

Thus when a person is suffering from liver damage, is unable to speak except by slurring his speech and feels ill, does society treat him as a sick person or as a drunk? For the argument over whether alcoholism is a disease is an argument over what is to be socially recognised as sickness. Similarly, a person may have no objective damage that can be detected, have clear signs of impaired functioning, but feel no unease at all. In such a case, should he be classed as a psychotic or is he merely not conforming to the rules of society. This is no abstract argument as the psychiatric wards in the USSR testify. There is, in short, wide variation in what is recognised as sickness: different subgroups within society (see Hessler et al., 1975) and different societies label the same 'objective' organic changes as sickness, crime, witchcraft or moral failing. For example, in Hong Kong physical and medical remedies are used to treat Haak-ts'an, which can be translated as 'injury by fright', while measles is treated by actions which suggest it is seen not as a disease but as a temporary social condition (see Topley, 1970).

Despite these wide variations in the criteria of affliction, it has been possible to develop a sociological concept of 'sickness' (i.e. the social recognition of organic or psychological change) that appears applicable to all cultures, although its referent may well be different in different cultures. Such a definition is given by Young (1976) when he defines sickness as

a kind of behaviour which would be socially unacceptable (because it involves withdrawal from customary responsibilities) if it were not that some means of exculpation is always provided. Exculpation usually takes place through notions of biophysical determinism...sometimes through the actions of agencies which are external to the sick person, but always by some mechanism which removes or distances the responsibility for the sick person's behaviour from his volition.

In short the sick person cannot be blamed for he does not have full control of himself - he has lost some will.

Treating 'sickness' as a cultural label has meant that sociologists have been able to analyse it in the same manner they use for analysing other cultural labels such as social class, gender or ethnicity. Similarly, they have been able to analyse the institution of healing in the same way they analyse such institutions as the family, religion or politics. Thus healing has been analysed as a 'message system' carrying messages about social and physical reality just as do other message systems such as ritual[1]. It has also been analysed as an institution fulfilling 'functions' in the society in which it operates, such as binding together a rural community or providing a means of acculturation for peasants flocking into the cities of the developing world (see Clark, 1970; Lieban, 1965, 1966, 1967; Press, 1969, 1971, 1978; Romano, 1965).

However interesting such accounts are, and they are fascinating, they do not provide an answer to the question of how healing works except to argue that it works by changing the cultural label, i.e. they argue that healers (in contrast to doctors) treat 'sickness', the social recognition of organic or psychological change, and not 'disease', the organic change. Such treatment of 'sickness' may affect 'illness' (the patient's unease) by naming the affliction the individual is suffering from and providing him with a set of beliefs and behaviours that purport to control it (see Eisenberg, 1977; Frankenberg and Leeson, 1976; Kleinman, 1973; Kleinman and Sung, 1976; Lewis, 1975). This is the import of work[2] which suggests that native healers are always successful because what they are engaged in is not cure of objective physiological states but changes in cultural labels. Given that both healer and client understand and believe in the techniques that change cultural labels, this is always a successful task. What is being suggested is that healing works because it defines affliction as a cultural rather than a physiological event and modifies cultural labels.

However, there is ample evidence that healing is concerned

not only with sickness (the social recognition of affliction) but also with disease (organic change), and there is some evidence - especially well-documented at Lourdes - that healing produces organic change. Given this evidence, it is no longer adequate sociology to treat man as an organic machine (to be studied by doctors) with feelings (to be studied by psychologists), who applies labels to his behaviour (to be studied by sociologists)[3]. A new model of man is required that does not treat man as a 'disembodied' self. That model must, if it is to be useful for looking at healing, include not only culture but also body and mind as social constructs, in part at least. I shall be spending the next several pages in constructing such a model, to which I give the name 'identity', and in citing evidence that supports such a model. I shall then go on to argue that healing is a process which seeks to change a person's identity through methods which I call 'transformation' and 'transcendence'. The difficulty with using the concept of identity is that it immediately plunges one into a philosophical morass. Before I begin to pick my way through this morass, it is important to reiterate that I am not engaged in a philosophical task. I am interested not in the ultimate truth of statements about soul, body, mind, spirit and identity, but in the construction of a model of identity that is to be judged on its utility as a heuristic device, a tool for explanation, not on its ultimate truth or falsity.

IDENTITY

Philosophical concern with identity centres around the concepts of 'mind' and 'body'[4]. This concern can be expressed as two problems: (1) the problem of ontology. How many different kinds of things are there in the world? Is the mind a different type of thing than the body? (2) The problem of epistemology. How do we know anything? How do we know what we know? It is important to realise that in this debate 'mind' is not the same as 'brain'. The brain is seen as a material thing, part of the body. Answers to the first question, how many different kinds of things are there in the world, are usually expressed as a debate between monism and dualism - between those who believe there is only one entity and those who believe there are two entities. Answers to the second question, how do we know anything, are usually expressed as a debate between positivism and idealism - between those who believe the only way we can know things is through our senses and those who believe the only things we can be sure of knowing are in our own mind.

When we look at the monist/dualist debate, it becomes obvious that it cannot be clearly separated from the epistemological debate. Those who believe that there is only one entity, the monists, can take several positions. They can argue that everything is mental and take up an idealist position (e.g. Hegel), or they can argue that nothing is mental, everything is physical, and take up a materialist position (e.g. Skinner). Alternatively, they can argue that the mental and the physical are just different aspects of the one entity (e.g. Spinoza, Bateson), i.e. that the person is a cybernetic system. Or they can argue that mind is an emergent property of the brain just as, for example, society is an emergent property of individuals (e.g. Bindra, Wilkes). Similarly, there are a variety of dualist positions ranging from those who see the physical as controlled by the mind (e.g. Plato, Thomas Aquinas) to those who see them as in interaction (e.g. Descartes).

How can we resolve this debate? Can it be resolved? There are certainly those who think it is insoluble. For my part the debate can be resolved sufficiently for my heuristic purposes by an examination of the evidence from neurobiology. There are three sets of data available from neurobiologists which appear to help in this resolution. Firstly there is the evidence from a variety of sources that behaviour can be affected by changes in the body chemistry and/or electrical stimulation (see. e.g. Black, 1969; Delgado, 1969; Rosenfeld, 1975). Now one of the features of the notion of 'mind' is that ideas are non-material, yet it seems the psychotropic drugs can change ideas. This would suggest that the idealists are wrong. Secondly there is the evidence (summarised in Stent, 1978) that sensory impressions do not arrive in the brain directly from the outside world. The receptors of the body, because of the way they are constructed[5], filter out certain sensory impressions and pass on only some of the many inputs to which the individual is exposed. This would suggest the positivists are wrong. Thirdly there is the data from split-brain research (Bindra (1976) reports this research). Here, for clinical reasons, a set of patients had the two halves of their brain separated by cutting the tissue joining them. These patients then exhibited the phenomena of two 'minds'. Because only one-half of the brain (normally the left) is capable of speech, when, in an experimental situation, a split-brain patient is shown one word with his right eye and a different word with his left eye, he only reports the word seen by his right eye. This means that information given to such a patient in one hemisphere is not transferred to the other. There is thus no overall 'mind', only a physical brain (or in this case brains).

What does this neurobiological data mean for the mind/body debate? It means that idealist explanations are untenable, that positivists' explanations are untenable and finally that 'mind' as an immaterial organiser and locus of experience does not appear to exist. The only way these apparent philosophical contradictions can be reconciled is (a) to abandon the notion of mind and (b) to suggest an alternative way of explaining perception, thought and behaviour. For Wilkes (1978) and Bindra (1976) this alternative notion is to posit a hierarchy of functions, in which higher functions have a reality greater than the parts which compose them.

This is a commonplace argument in sociology: society has a

reality independent of the individuals who compose it. This can be seen most obviously in terms of the fact that society contrives to operate after the death of individuals, and in the phenomena of language which exists independently of any one individual speaker. But this does not lead sociologists to posit an immaterial 'social mind' to explain the operation of society. Such reification is eschewed in favour of an explanation that sees the operation of society as a result of the complexity of the interrelationship between individuals, a complexity that has a different mode of operation than the individuals who create it. Similarly, Wilkes and Bindra argue that there is no need to posit a real immaterial mind; mental functions are emergent functions which have a different mode of operation than the individual neurological events that create them. 'Mind' exists as 'society' exists but it exists as a way of explaining reality. It is an analytic device, not a real thing. The problems arise when people use the concept of 'mind' as a cause of events rather than using it as a convenient way of describing them.

If, however, we abandon the notion of an immanent mind with which the individual is born and see him as a neurological complex, then where does our conception of identity come from? Why do we distinguish ourselves as independent entities with an inside and an outside? Why do we feel that we continue the same being from one situation to another? The answers to these questions are I believe sociological rather than philosophical. We develop our awareness of ourselves as separate beings, continuous over time, from the processes we undergo and continue to undergo as we grow up. The implication of this, and it is to this point that my argument leads, is that if we change the process we change the identity. This is what is healing is doing.

My model [6] of this process starts with the baby at birth. At this time it has no concept of itself at all. There is no reason why it should. For the first months of its life it has been part of another person, little different in that respect than a stomach, and we do not expect a stomach to have a sense of identity. At this stage the child has no identity, makes no distinction between itself and its environment. It has no boundary [7]. Yet after birth it quickly develops the idea of boundary, the unverbalised feeling that 'this is me, this is not me', even without the concepts to symbolically represent that feeling. It develops that awareness from the actions of others towards it, particularly the actions of feeding and touch, which are, significantly, closely interrelated. Touch, in fact, may even be more important than feeding. When the Harlows presented a group of infant monkeys with dummy surrogate parents, they chose the dummy that had cloth in preference to the one that had food (reported in Becker, 1971). It is interesting, in this respect, to note that touch is the only sense in which all the body is represented (Gray Walter, 1953). From touch and feeding the child derives a boundary, a positive identity of itself as an individual. This constitutes the first of our identities in this model. (By distinguishing four identities it is not being suggested that an individual actually possesses four separate identities. These distinctions are analytic not real. In fact identity in this model is a process best expressed as a verb, not the noun our language forces us to use. I shall return to this point later.) The second identity developed by the child is an active one. It experiments within the world, it moves its limbs, its mouth and its bowels and from this derives an active sense of self - not I am, but I can - 'I can move that object, I can scream, I can move that arm.' It does not, of course, say these things because it has, as yet, no symbols with which to do so. Nonetheless even at this stage it is a complex being with two analytically distinguishable identities: a passive bodily identity and an active bodily identity.

It is the interaction between these two identities which acts as a lever to move the child onto the next stage in its development - the stage in which it takes into itself the demands of its trainers. The child notes that some of the objects around it react to its actions, e.g. they often stop it doing things. Importantly they are the objects on which it depends for food and touch, on which it depends for the maintenance of its first passive bodily identity. It is in a dilemma. As an active being it wishes to do certain things, but if it does them it displeases those who provided and continue to provide it with its first passive identity (for identity is not a once and for all thing, it has to be continually re-affirmed). It resolves the dilemma by taking into itself, internalising, the demands of its trainers. No longer does it want to do things that threaten its primary passive identity, it wants to do what its trainers want it to do. It has become socialised. In Freudian terms it has acquired a super-ego; in behaviourist terms it has been conditioned. The active identity is directed along certain channels so that its acts are acceptable to its trainers.

The organism, as it has been depicted so far, could have been any animal. The next stage takes the development of the child outside the animal kingdom. It reacts not just to the actions of its trainers but to their vocalisations. Even at this stage it appears no different than a trained animal. The difference lies in the fact that it does not just react to the vocalisations but understands them. It learns to understand the speech. The process is mysterious. Arguments rage in linguistics about whether the understanding of language is instinctual or social. The fact is it happens and it makes the child human and not animal. (See Lyons's (1970) discussion of Chomsky.) Words give others control over him. They divide up reality in such a way that they guide the process of thinking and channel it along set lines. They lead the individual to think about the world in a similar way to others of his family, tribe and nation. In particular he learns such basic conceptual frameworks as those of space and time. He becomes human. His human identity is an important and precious thing and this importance is celebrated by presenting him with a symbol - a name. One can see why naming ceremonies are such an important event in all societies and why names are often secret, for in them lies the social, human, identity of the person named. The child is of course not just talked at. He does not just acquire a passive human identity. He too learns to talk and derives an identity as an active symbol user. The manipulation of words, or more correctly the manipulation of meaning, gives him a control over his world that is both more far-reaching and more subtle than any physical exercise of his body could achieve for him.

The model of man is now complete. Man is seen as possessing four analytically distinguishable identities:

(1) a primary passive identity as a
    bounded body   )
) 'animal' identity
(2) an active bodily identity   )

(3) a passive identity as a receiver   )
    of symbols   )
) 'social' identity
(4) an active identity as a user of   )
    symbols   )

There is nothing radically new in this model of identity, most of the ideas underlying it have been expressed before. The idea that an individual's identity is constructed in interaction with others is the main theme in G.H. Mead's work (1970). Similarly Laing (1971) argues that 'one's first social identity is conferred on one. We learn to be whom we are told we are.' Laing also argues the existentialist philosophic position that we are continually in the process of 'becoming'. Our identity is not fixed but continually being re-affirmed or disconfirmed in interaction with others. As I suggested earlier, identity is a process not a thing. What is new in this model is that this conception of the creation of identity is not restricted to social identity but extended to bodily identity also. Mead was a philosopher and was concerned with mental constructs. His concept of identity creation was thus one of symbolic interaction; my concept is one of interaction that is physical as well as interaction in terms of symbols.

My argument is that there remains only one identity. This means that the social identity and the physical identity are interlinked, that the socially constructed identities and the physically constructed identities are closely interrelated. There is some evidence and some argument that supports this contention. Manning and Fabrega (1973) argue that the very idea of a separate social identity (or 'mind') and body is itself a product of a particular social structure. In traditional societies the (social) self, the body, interpersonal relations and nature are seen in continuity; the microcosm reflects the macrocosm. This view of the world is familiar to us from Shakespeare's plays where the storms and tempests portend disorder in the social world, and is explained in detail in Keith Thomas's excellent book (1973). With the development of complex societies, and in particular with urbanisation, the individual is constantly forced into new situations. His experience is no longer continuous and he has to adjust. One adjustment is to see the self as remaining true to itself when acting in the correct manner in each situation although this implies behaving differently in different situations. This has been the traditional Japanese response. One western response has been to conceive of the self as having a continuity in a fundamental self, a conscience, an authentic self which is the core being, acting regardless of situation (Reisman et al., 1950; Turner, 1976). Another western response has been to clearly distinguish the body, which remains the same in each situation, from the mind, which can change as the situation changes. Much of western dramatic literature is concerned with the conjunction of these two responses, with ethical value being placed on acting according to 'conscience', the first rather than the second response.

Whether or not the distinction between the body and the social self is an historical accident it remains true that they are closely related. First there is the clear evidence from clinical data on amputations that a change in the body leads to a change in the self-identity of an individual. The evidence suggests that certain parts of the body are more central than others in this respect; the face, the torso (and for women the breasts) are more important than appendages (Lipowski 1969; Renneker and Cutler, 1952; Sutherland and Orback 1953; Wright, 1960). Secondly there is evidence from Fisher and Cleveland's (1968) extensive work that a person's self-identity contains an element they call 'body-image' and that the type of body image held is related to disease patterns. They show specifically that people with strong perceptions of the body boundary, called 'high barrier', develop exterior psychosomatic symptoms such as arthritis and dermatitis significantly more than those with a low barrier. Concomitantly 'low barrier' individuals develop interior symptoms such as stomach pains and colitis more often than those with 'high barriers'. Thus, just as the first set of evidence, derived from amputation, suggests that changes in the body produce changes in self-image, the second set, derived from Fisher and Cleveland's work, suggests that change in self-image (for 'body image' is not a physical thing) can produce changes in the body. As Rosenfeld (1975) expresses it: 'mind and matter, brain and behaviour, are one. They can be thought of and dealt with separately, as an artifice for man's convenience, but in reality they are inseparable. In this scheme of things, changes in the mental sphere are never unaccompanied by changes in the physical.'

What does this imply for healing? After all it was for an exploration of healing that the model was constructed in the first place. To answer this question we have to look at another implication of the model. The model sees the process

121

of constructing an identity as one conducted in interaction with other people. It also sees this process as necessarily never complete, always open-ended. Identity is not a fixed thing but a process in which the reactions of other people sustain our identity or deny it. Couple this fact with the argument in the previous paragraph that identity is composed of body and culturally created identity intimately interlinked and the relevance to healing becomes clear. Identity is created and sustained by social interaction. A change in social interaction produces a change in identity, and the body is included in the term identity. There is, in fact, already extensive evidence that changes in the social environment produce changes in bodily states. Chertok (1969) argues that a breakdown in interpersonal relationships leads to illness and re-establishment of such relationships produces health, and Kimball (1970) summarises the evidence in support of this contention.

Even stronger support comes from the work on stress. It has long been known that stress can cause disease. The most widely publicised example is the duodenal ulcer. Even the mechanisms by which this effect occurs have been known for some time. The central nervous system, by way of the hypothalamus, and the autonomic nervous system, by way of the production of adrenalin, have profound effects upon the body. Both nervous systems can be changed in their operations by emotions (Abrahamson and Pezet, 1951; Black, 1968) and emotions are socially created and defined states[8]. What recent research seems to suggest is that people whom one would expect to be suffering similar stress because they are undergoing similar stress-producing disruptions and changes in their lives react very differently. The difference in susceptibility to illness and to the development of disease seem not to be related to their physiological state. In fact Cobb (1976) presents clear evidence that they are related to social support. Those people who have a lot of stressful changes in their life, but have some social support, are less likely to get ill and more likely to get better if they are ill than those without such support:

> adequate social support can protect people in crisis from a wide variety of pathological states: from low birth weight to death, from arthritis through tuberculosis to depression, alcoholism and to other psychiatric illness. Furthermore social support can reduce the amount of medication required and accelerate recovery and facilitate compliance with prescribed medical regimens...The hypothesis is strong, but as far as I know untested, that social support facilitates identity change, which in turn, facilitates role change (from a sick role to a healthy role).

TRANSFORMATION

As I argued at the beginning of this chapter most

anthropological and sociological accounts of healing concentrate on the techniques, procedures and social rituals whereby societies redefine sickness. Such studies on primitive societies and peasant societies[9] generally conclude that the healing process is as much concerned with the cure of the society as it is with the cure of the patients. Healing is seen as a means of re-integrating a society disrupted by the illness of one of its members rather than a means of re-integrating the individual, regardless of society. The healing is seen to be complete when the individual is re-integrated into the society, regardless of his state of awareness of his bodily state and regardless of the bodily state itself. Such explanations are inadequate because they abdicate the sociologist's responsibility to find sociological explanations and they are inadequate because they fail to take into account the patient's criteria of success. If the patient does not feel better, if they are not healed of their 'illness', then they, and other members of their society, are not willing to see the healing of their 'sickness' as sufficient. It is important therefore that the sociologist should provide a sociological account not only of the healing process that produces a healing of sickness - the cultural label - but also one that produces an account of the healing process that produces a healing of illness - the patient's feelings. Such an account is provided by the argument that people who feel ill are taken through a process that transforms their identity so that they feel well.

The process starts with a person approaching a healer because they are suffering from an affliction. They feel a pain or suffer a disability either of which makes it difficult for them to continue acting in their normal manner. The afflicted person turns in upon himself and centres his attention upon the state of his body or his mind so that the affliction becomes a major factor in his life (Lederer, 1965; Lipowski, 1969). In turn, because he is behaving differently, others act toward him differently (Cruickshank, 1948; Ladieu et al., 1948; White et al., 1948). All afflictions have this effect. They disrupt the plans of people for tomorrow; normal life has to be reorganised. They change the pattern of social relations people are accustomed to, for example by making it difficult or impossible to go to work and interact with workmates. They change the body image people hold. They reduce autonomy of action (Bernard, 1975). These effects of affliction are particularly pronounced amongst the clients of marginal healers for such clients commonly have afflictions which are considered incurable, chronic or mental, any of which radically alters the behaviour of others toward the individual. Acute short-term disease has only a limited effect on a person's identity, but chronic and mental afflictions have a profound effect (Field, 1976). This is especially true if these afflictions carry a social stigma (Goffman, 1968). The clients of marginal healers have these particular types of afflictions because people normally only turn to marginal healers as a last resort, when orthodox

medicine has failed them[10], and orthodox medicine is least
successful with these types of affliction. Such afflictions
are extremely common, e.g. cardiovascular disorders,
respiratory disease, muscular sketetal diseases such as
arthritis, and mental and nervous diseases, cause between
them the most lost working days in Britain (Tuckett, 1976).
Such afflictions respond to management rather than crisis
intervention and they are also the diseases that benefit
from any type of treatment (Maclean, 1971).

The treatment that chronic or mental sufferers do receive
from marginal healers is concerned with changing the
identity of the individual. Marginal healing concentrates
upon healing the person not the disease. This is true of
'eastern' healers. Christian healers and radionic healers:

> We view the person as a process containing active and
> passive elements. Disease is disharmony. Treatment
> therefore is to restore harmony, to change the
> process not to treat an organ. ('Eastern' healer)

> It has to be recognised that man is a unity in which
> the whole person must be treated. (Christian healer -
> a Burrswood pamphlet)

> Radionics is an entelechtic holistic approach to
> healing; it is above all concerned with the total
> man. (Radionics pamphlet)

In this respect they differ from doctors, who concentrate
upon 'disease' - organic change. They also differ from
healers in primitive and peasant societies, who concentrate
upon 'sickness' - the social definition of affliction. A
concern with 'disease' leads to a focus on the patterns of
symptoms presented by an individual. A concern with
'sickness' leads to a concentration upon the patterns of
social stress which are focused on an individual. The first
leads to a therapy which mobilizes material forces to cure
the individual independently of his will. The second leads
to a therapy which mobilises social forces to cure the
individual, equally independently of his will. Marginal
healers in modern society, by contrast, focus upon the
individual and his feelings ('illness') and their therapy
requires the co-operation of the individual. What is
involved in their therapy is a complex process of coaching
(see Strauss, 1959) whereby the individual abandons his old
identity as an afflicted individual subject to his
affliction and takes on a new identity as an individual who
controls his affliction. He moves from a passive identity to
an active identity. It is as though an affliction is a
powerful wave before which the individual is helpless. It
sweeps away his old life and takes away his will. Healers,
by coaching, teach the individual to ride the wave, to use
this powerful force. The individual may even exploit the
force of the wave to develop skills (of self-development) of
which he would not otherwise be aware, so that the wave is
seen, in part, as a blessing rather than an unmitigated
disaster.

How is this change achieved? It is achieved over a period of time by an interaction between the healer and the client in which the healer treats the client as a worthy individual. This is not a simple matter of the healer telling the client that he is important as an individual but a complex social process. One vital element in this process is that the client sees the healer as authoritative[11]. It is no use anyone telling an afflicted individual that they are worthy if the views do not carry any weight; the healer has to be important enough so that his views matter. This is one purpose of the testimonials that all healers provide for their clients at some stage in their treatment. A man who has healed before can heal again. More importantly, however, healers tap a symbol system and a language that already has an air of authority. For some healers this is religion and they use the language and symbols of religion. For others it is science and they use the language and symbols of science[12]. For others both symbol systems are called into play, e.g. Harry Edwards wore a white coat, talked of energy, but saw his healing power as coming ultimately from God, and he conducted his healing in a room with an altar and a cross. An important element in the construction of authority for many healers is that their authority lies outside themselves with God. If God is doing the healing then his authority is absolute (Kiev, 1966b; Mischel, 1959). The 'trickery' of psychic surgeons is also a means of gaining authority. If such people can make incisions with their bare hands then anything is possible to them (Eliade, 1964). In addition to this legitimizing of authority, healers in Britain also gain authority from their (presumed) upper-class background, signalled by their speech, or from their association with upper-class patrons[13]. Most of the healers I studied were male and the majority of their clients were female, both healer and client normally being of a generation in which the differences between the sexes were accepted as hierarchical. Finally, all the healers act with authority in their interpersonal relationships. On meeting healers one is struck immediately by the manner in which they establish an imposing presence on the relationship in a way which is dominant without being domineering. The lecture given to students at the college of healing outlined this aspect of their role very clearly (see p. 93).

This construction of an authoritative presence continues throughout the therapeutic process. It is not a once and for all event although first impressions are obviously important and the clothes of the healer and the props of his consulting room play an important role in this first impression. The first contact between healer and client is not just one where the healer establishes his authority, it is also one where the healer begins to treat the individual with respect. One of the first tasks of most healers is to elicit from the client what is wrong with them. They allow and encourage the client to talk about themselves, and importantly, they pay attention to the client's own words. For example, the cymatic practitioner and the Ramana Health

Centre both have forms that allow patients to express their problems in their own words[14].

In so doing they are implying that what the client says is important and hence the client is worthy of attention as an individual. This does not mean that they necessarily give the client personal attention but that they give attention to the person as an individual. They are concerned not with finding out a set of symptoms from which they can diagnose, as a doctor is, but with finding out what sort of individual a person is so that they can treat. Their mode of communication is therefore different from that of a doctor. A doctor initiates his consultation by an open question, 'How are you?' but does not expect a full answer, only a starting-point from which he can initiate further questions to solve a diagnostic puzzle (Coulthardt and Ashby, 1976). A healer, although he initiates his consultation in the same way, does expect a full answer and expects to spend most of his first consultation with a patient listening rather than questioning. Thus, even at this early stage in the therapeutic process, the client is the active individual and the healer the passive one. As Press (1978) says, 'curers, as opposed to physicians, take their cues from patients...and thus offer a guarantee that the patient's peculiar anxieties and sick role preference will be validated'. Not surprisingly this art of sympathetic listening is valued by healers:

> It's personal contact that is vital. You have to make contact quickly - like a confidence trickster, the same skills. You listen, but first you've got to get them to talk[15].

It is valued as a means of diagnosis:

> Ask what's wrong, not push it too far or they might clam up...At the same time form some opinion on the way they sit, the way they hold their hands, the way they use their eyes. (See Chapter 5)

and it is also valued as a mode of therapy:

> (Clients) are usually treated with such a great amount of detachment by other people, other places they've had treatment, they're treated so much as numbers...the fact that you're going to treat them entirely as an individual for half an hour, your undivided attention (is important). (See Chapter 5)

In short, by listening to them talk about themselves, by allowing them to express themselves in their own words, by giving their clients time, healers relate to them as worthy individuals. As one healer succinctly put it 'you never laugh at a patient'. Given this fact it is hardly surprising that their clients see their healers as having empathy, genuineness, non-possessive warmth, technical competence and strong interpersonal attributes (reported by Parker and Tupling, 1976).

Healers not only act passively with their clients to signal to them their worth, they also engage in behaviour that actively signals that worth. One technique employed is to reflect back to the client a positive image of himself. The technique of listening goes further than merely giving the client the opportunity to be active, it actually forces an active identity upon the client.

> if one of the...county set comes in - you know, yacht club, country club, got their own boats...you must immediately start talking on that level...adapting your own personality.

> Be a reflection of the person you're treating...to be a more reliable, more secure part of themselves...So you are the rock, absolutely dependable, absolutely competent, absolutely sure of everything you do and as you're reflecting them they too can become sure of themselves. (See Chapter 5)

It is not just through words that this new identity is built up, however. It is also achieved by what Goffman (1956) called 'presentational rituals'. There is an interesting distinction to be made here. Goffman distinguishes two modes of demonstrating respect or, as he calls it, deference. The first mode he calls 'avoidance rituals' and these consist of demonstrating respect by keeping one's distance, respecting privacy. The second mode, 'presentational rituals', demonstrates respect by invading privacy. I suggest that 'avoidance rituals' are used when one wishes to show respect to a role, including in the category role as well as such obvious roles as president or priest, the role of person. In contrast, 'presentational rituals' are utilised whenever one wishes to show respect not to a role but to an individual. Many people act towards the sick as a category, a role - sick person - and show deference to that category by keeping their distance, speaking in special hushed tones, avoiding the use of certain words (e.g. the word 'see' with a blind person) and deliberately not looking at their affliction if it is visible, in short behaving in the manner so ably described by Goffman (1968) when discussing stigma. In contrast healers act toward the sick as individuals, showing respect to the individual not the category.

The time many healers give to their clients is also important here because the more interaction that is undertaken the more difficult it is to treat the person you are interacting with in terms of their role rather than their individuality. Anybody who has worked with disfigured or disabled people for any length of time soon fails to see the disfigurement and sees only the individual. The actual 'presentational rituals' that Goffman distinguished were the use of first names, the proffering of small services and aid, invitations to come on outings, salutations and touch. All of these rituals were used by the healers studied, and though each appears only a minor act in itself, in total they express the important fact that healers were treating individuals with respect. These rituals were particularly evident at Lourdes (see Chapter 3) where the roles of brancadier and lady helper consisted precisely of these presentational rituals. Salutations are particularly important in the coaching relationship that is built up between healer and client for they act as markers of progress, 'benchmarks' (Roth, 1963), which signal to healer and client how far the client has progressed. By noticing and commenting upon changes in the client the healer signals that he is interested in the client as an individual. By noticing and commenting only upon positive changes in the client, the healer provides the client with cues as to the appropriate demeanour of a healthy identity: 'We never tell people they're not getting better. You go to a doctor to get tablets, you go to a healer to get well[16].' Touch too is very important. It breaks down the egocentric isolation of the sick person (see Skultans, 1974) and in addition it is related to body boundaries and basic animal identities (a point that will be returned to later when discussing transcendence).

In addition all healers require of their clients that they take an active part in the healing process. As Frank (1963, p.98) says:

All methods of promoting healing...through personal influence seem to require the object of the influence to participate actively in the proceedings... Moreover, characteristically, the nature of the activities is not completely prescribed so that he must take some initiative. The contents of his confession, for example...are always up to him.

Amongst the healers I studied there was a similar emphasis upon the client ultimately taking responsibility for his own health. Those doctors sympathetic to alternative medicine are most active in promoting this point of view, but it is a view widely held amongst healers, e.g. a Burrswood pamphlet (Chapter 3) states 'The patient must be convinced that he need not be limited by his past. He must be helped to become responsible.' Such a demand for active participation not only avoids the production of a passive individual, rather than the active individual healers are trying to produce, it also makes a change in the individual's identity more likely to be sustained: the greater the difficulties encountered, the greater the trials undergone and so the more active the commitment required, the more likely that a new identity will be sustained.

Sustaining the new active identity is done in a variety of ways. As one healer[17], said, 'I give them something to structure their lives around, it varies from person to person.' It varies not only from person to person but also from healer to healer. Typically, healers admonish their clients to maintain the new body posture or the better movement achieved by healing. They suggest a new diet, a new life style. They give the client new mental or physical

exercises. In addition, to prevent backsliding and to
encourage the client to maintain the new mode of life, they
ask for progress reports or names to be entered on a
thanksgiving list[18]. Typical of such activities is the
description of a special cancer treatment in a pamphlet
distributed by Harry Edwards:

> In the beginning we show the patient how to lose all
> fear of cancer. He is encouraged to think positively
> and to look ahead as the body's health and resistance
> is built up...The patient is requested to enter into
> a thirty minute meditation each day. We are insistent
> about this. We supply printed directions to cover
> all these matters. Lastly a weekly report is to be
> sent to the healer who answers each letter
> personally...Special healing sessions are held
> monthly to which all patients are invited.

The necessity to analyse the elements in the process of
losing an old identity and learning a new identity should
not be allowed to divert attention from the fact that what
is occurring is a process. The elements in the process are
interlinked and feed back one upon another. An example
already mentioned in discussing Lourdes illustrates this
point. Two of the sick pilgrims, Joan and Marie, were
paraplegics. Joan was very withdrawn: at home she spent her
days alone in a small room watching television, on the
pilgrimage she was further alienated by being a working-
class non-Catholic amongst upper-class Catholics. Marie, by
contrast, was extremely outgoing: she was married to a
fellow member of a home for paraplegics and was a leader in
the home amongst its inmates, she was also a Catholic and
classless (her Canadian upbringing). At the beginning of the
week of pilgrimage the prognosis, therefore, looked much
better for Marie. She was seeking interaction while Joan was
repudiating it. The odds on improvement seemed biased
towards Marie. However, this was not what happened. Marie
insisted on clinging to her old identity and frequently
talked about her spouse and her important position in the
home for paraplegics. Joan, on the other hand, was gradually
drawn out of her shell by the helpers who picked out the one
aspect of her identity that singled her out. She liked as
she put it 'an occasional glass of stout'. This was built up
in interaction so that it became an integral part of a new
identity as a working-class woman fond of a laugh and a
drink, an identity she gradually adopted as her own. For the
helpers this change brought its own rewards. Their
interaction with Joan brought about a measurable change in
her attitude and demeanour, giving them immense
satisfaction, and the identity she developed made her fun to
be with. Thus by the end of the pilgrimage week it was Joan
who was the life and soul of the party and Marie was left,
if not isolated, at least somewhat set apart. Joan also
became physically better, able to hold a glass of stout by
herself, stout playing an important part of her new
identity. Marie, on the other hand, declared she hadn't
enjoyed Lourdes at all and certainly wouldn't come again.

Healers in general are aware that clients sometimes insist on clinging to their old identities and that some clients, in fact, may insist on clinging to the identity of a sick person and like institutionalised prisoners be loath to step outside it: 'Out of every ten people, four drop out, four keep coming until we've mutually agreed we've done all we can. These are the successful. Two are more neurotic, who you could continue to see for life, and whom the unscrupulous could rob for life[17].'

In this section of the chapter I have argued that the healing which most marginal healers are involved in for most of the time is a process of transforming the identity of the afflicted individual. The idea of healing as a learning process has been discussed in the sociological literature before (see Frank, 1963; Kiev, 1966b; Kleinman and Sung, 1976) and the idea of healing as a transformation from a passive to an active identity forms the substance of many arguments about healing as a rite of passage (see e.g. Turner, 1963 and 1968). What is new in this concept is that the transformation of identity is seen to be achieved by means other than ritual, namely through a process of coaching.

This is the most common form of healing and it is a long drawn-out process which is not spectacular or miraculous. Harry Edwards, for example, who actually has had cripples walk off the stage after his treatment, says: 'All spiritual healing is a gradual process. Sensational or "miracle" healings do take place on occasion, but they are an exception to the general rule.'

A point echoed by McNutt (1974, p.125) when he states that 'Many healings are progressive and require the continued support of a Christian community.' The aim of the healer is to move the client from a position where he is dominated by his affliction and is passive in the face of it to a position where he dominates his affliction and is active in his life. This does not mean that the disease is cured. The individual can be healed if he incorporates the illness as part of his identity and adopts it as a means of developing his identity. In this fashion the illness is no longer seen as an externally imposed affliction to be resented but as part of the self to be exploited. In its extreme form this view may even appear to be a celebration of sickness: 'If we don't suffer enough it is because we are not worthy. We must regard those who suffer more with reverence and a certain awe. You have the privilege of suffering. You are suffering for us[19]'. It may be seen as a successful healing when a person dies, as long as they are in active control of their identity. This explains the apparently paradoxical statement that 'the ministry of healing seems to open the way to a marvellous and radiant death'.

However, if healing is generally a process of coaching an individual from a passive to an active identity it still remains true that occasionally it is more than that. There are occasional 'miracles', occasional 'spontaneous' cures. How can they be explained? Well, if most healing can be seen as a transformation of <u>social</u> identity, in terms of the model of identity presented earlier, then miraculous healings can be seen as transcendence of <u>animal</u> identities in addition to the transformation of social identity and this is the subject of the next section.

TRANSCENDENCE

It seems reasonable that sociology may be able to explain changes in 'sickness' as sickness is after all socially defined. It may even be possible that sociology can provide an explanation for healing of 'illness', for, one can argue, the perception of oneself is constructed in social interaction. But it seems highly improbable that sociology can provide an explanation for the healing of 'disease' for disease is by this definition a bodily state. How can immaterial social forces produce changes in a material being? How they may do so is the subject of this section of the chapter. It only seems an insuperable problem if the body is seen as in some sense independent of the symbolic environment in which it exists. I have already argued in constructing my model of 'identity' that this is not the case. Bodily identity is, in part, a social construction. If this is so it can be reconstructed by manipulation of the social world. There is extensive evidence that this does occur. Wolf (1959) in his early study of the placebo effect came to the conclusion that 'the mechanisms of the human body are capable of reacting not only to direct physical and chemical stimulation but also to symbolic stimuli, words and events which have somehow acquired special meaning for the individual'.

A good account of such a reaction is given by Klopfer (1957) describing a Mr Wright who was suffering from advanced cancer. He was not expected to live more than a month but he heard of a new drug that was expected to cure cancer. He pestered his doctor for this drug although it was only being tried out on patients with a prognosis of at least three months life. After a few days on the drug his tumours had shrunk to half their original size and in ten days he was discharged. Within two months reports appeared that the drug did not work and he relapsed. His doctor then (deliberately lying) informed him that the reports were wrong and that he had relapsed because the drug had deteriorated on the shelf, a new batch would soon put him right. He then gave him an injection of water. Once again the tumours disappeared and he left the hospital. He finally died several months later when a report of the American Medical Association announced that the drug was worthless.

Anecdotes such as this are not conclusive evidence of the effect of social context on the physical body but coupled with the detailed experimental evidence from researchers such as Wolf they are strongly suggestive. In addition there is a theoretical framework into which such evidence can be fitted. Developed in research on the effects of electrical and chemical stimulation of the brain this model sees the individual as a construction of the inputs into him: 'each person is a transitory composite of materials borrowed from the environment' (Delgado, 1969, p.56). It follows from this model that a change in input will produce a change in identity: 'mind and matter, brain and behaviour are one. They can be thought of and dealt with separately as an artifice for man's convenience, but in reality they are inseparable. In this scheme of things, changes in the mental sphere are never unaccompanied by changes in the physical' (Rosenfeld, 1975. p.212). This is already well accepted for explaining disease. Tucket (1976, p.386) summarises the extensive evidence for this when he says 'the cause of many diseases...can be found in a complex chain of interaction between "whole" humans and their physical and social environment that gives individuals identity and meaning.' What I want to argue here is that what is true as an explanation of disease may be equally true as an explanation of healing. If a change in the social environment can produce a change in the body so that it malfunctions, a change in the social environment may restore its functioning. Sociologists have for too long viewed the self as 'disembodied' (the phrase comes from Manning and Fabrega (1973)). It is time to construct a sociological account of man that takes into account his physical as well as his mental and social nature.

If changes in the physical body can be achieved by changes in input, what is the mechanism of that process? A definitive answer cannot be given without the co-operation of physiologists, psychologists and sociologists but some hints on the direction such research should take may be given. It seems, from the accounts of healing in which instantaneous cures occurred, that the individuals who were cured passed through a state of transcendence, e.g. Blanton (1940, p.359) describing a cure at Lourdes says:

> Now in this man and in similar sick people who go to Lourdes the important thing, we think, is that they have reached the limit of their emotional and physical capacities to adjust to the demands of their illness. For some reason...they cannot any longer accept life and yet they cannot quite accept death. Physically their libidinal drive is what may be termed reversible (because it does reverse itself) but their ego has reached a state of depletion so nearly complete that they themselves have not the capacity to reverse it. In our opinion, it is only when they have reached this state of complete surrender that they can be cured by such a transference - in this case to the Virgin Mother Mary who, they feel, intercedes for them with the Creator himself.

That is transcendence described in psychoanalytic terms - a

state of complete surrender in which the ego has reached a state of depletion. Described by those who have experienced such a state it is expressed in different language:

> I walked with a stick, had a disabled badge on my car, and frequently fell through lack of balance...they said they must pray for me...what they said I have no idea, as I suddenly relaxed in such a way as I had never done in the whole of my life. I found I could not open my eyes, and then suddenly a brilliant white light appeared in my eyes, followed by my breathing so deeply wihout any conscious effort on my part that I thought my lungs would burst. I then seemed to float in the air, talking all the while in a strange language which quickly released the blockage in my heart[20].

This state of transcendence or ecstasy is a state in which the individual gives up his will totally and loses his identity. I want to argue that it is in fact a return to the state before the individual had <u>any</u> identity at all, a return to the time even before the construction of an animal identity. In such a state the individual is a blank sheet on which a new identity can be constructed, a healthy identity. This conception of transcendence as a state of pre-individuality is not a new one. Martin Buber, the famous mystic and theologian, also perceived this state in the same way:

> Now from my own unforgettable experience I know well that there is a state in which the bonds of the personal nature of life seem to have fallen away from us and we experience an undivided unity. But I do not know what the soul willingly imagines and indeed is bound to imagine (mine too once did it) that in this I had attained to a union with the primal being or the godhead. This is an exaggeration no longer permitted to the responsible understanding. Responsible - that is, as a man holding his ground before reality - I can elicit from those experiences only that in them I reached an indifferentiable unity of myself without form or content. I may call this an original pre-biographical unity and suppose that it is hidden unchanged beneath all biographical change, all development and complication of soul. (1947, pp.24-5)

Accounts of such a state are usually expressed in mystical, poetic language for the experience is beyond words, being, as it is, an experience of a time when the individual has no identity from which he can comprehend the experience. Happold (1963) in his book has a collection of descriptions of this state, some invested with religious meaning, others having no meaning at all. Two examples may be useful here. The first is from the writing of Richard of St Victor who died in 1173:

The third degree of love is when the mind of a man is ravished into the abyss of divine light so that the soul, having forgotten all outward things, is altogether unaware of itself and passes out completely into its God. In this state it is wholly subdued, the host of carnal desires are deeply asleep and there is silence in heaven as it were for half an hour. And any suffering that is left is absorbed into glory. In this state while the soul is abstracted from itself, ravished into that secret place of divine refuge, when it is surrounded on every side by the divine fire of love, pierced to the core, set alight all about, then it sheds its very self altogether and puts on that divine life, and being wholly conformed to the beauty it has seen passes wholly into that glory.

The second is a secular account of a similar experience:

The thing happened one summer afternoon, on the school cricket field, while I was sitting on the grass, waiting my turn to bat. I was thinking about nothing in particular, merely enjoying the pleasures of midsummer idleness. Suddenly, and without warning something invisible seemed to be drawn across the sky, transforming the world about me into a kind of tent of concentrated and enhanced significance. What had merely been an outside became an inside. The objective was somehow transformed into a completely subjective fact, which was experienced as 'mine', but on a level where the word had no meaning; for 'I' was not longer the familiar ego. Nothing more can be said about the experience, it brought no accession of knowledge about anything except, very obscurely, the knower and his way of knowing. After a few minutes there was a 'return to normalcy'. The event made a deep impression on me at the time; but because it did not fit into any of the thought patterns - religious, philosophical, scientific - with which as a boy of fifteen I was familiar, it came to seem more and more anomalous, more and more irrelevant to 'real life', and was finally forgotten.

The state appears to be a property open to all men as it is a state that exists outside culture. (As Hine (1969) argues, for the associated state of glossolalia - speaking with tongues.) That does not mean however that cultures pay no attention to it. It is culturally interpreted but interpretation is widely variable. In our own society it is usually interpreted within the tradition of Christian mysticism although more recently the mysticism of Eastern religions has been invoked to express it. Amongst the Dinka as described by Lienhardt (1961) it is the central experience of their whole religious life. By contrast amongst the Kung bushmen the state is presumed to derive from men rather than spirits or the gods (Lee, 1968). The bushmen are particularly interesting in that they reverse the usual explanation of healing. In most cultures that produce a state of transcendence as part of a healing process the power that produces the healing is seen to come from outside man as a spiritual immaterial force. For the bushmen, on the other hand, it is disease that comes from the spirit realm and it is other men who provide the power to heal in the state of transcendence. Wherever the power comes from it is a state of transcendence that is common to these accounts.

Before looking at how this state is achieved it would be useful to summarize the characteristics of the transcendent state. Fortunately Ludwig (1968) provides such a summary and delineates the following features:

(1) alterations in thinking: the distinction between cause and effect is blurred and opposites can co-exist;
(2) disturbed time sense;
(3) loss of control;
(4) change in emotional expression: either an intense display of emotion or a lack of emotion;
(5) body image change: depersonalisation, dissolution of boundaries between the self and the world;
(6) perceptual distortion;
(7) change in significance: people give great significance to their experiences in this state;
(8) sense of the ineffable: the experience is beyond words;
(9) sense of rejuvenation, a sense of rebirth;
(10) hypersuggestibility.

How do people achieve such a state? How do people experience a state of non-identity? How are they literally born again? To achieve such a state requires a process that makes Goffman's (1971) description of the brutal identity stripping that occurs when people enter a total institution appear to be mild by comparison. On entering a total institution the individual loses only part of his cultural identity - his name and his possessions. He does not lose other aspects of his cultural identity, such as sex, nor does he lose his ability to be an active symbol manipulator. In fact much symbol use in total institutions by the inmates consists of profane language that asserts bodily functions (see Becker, 1971) and hence bodily identity. In the state described above, the state of transcendence, of ecstasy - the state of being outside oneself - the individual loses all identity, bodily identity as well as cultural identity.

This state is achieved by a series of techniques that break down the individual's bodily identity as well as their cultural identity, particularly with respect to such basic cultural concepts as space and time. However it is important to realise that though these techniques are applied to the individual, ultimately the individual has to be willing to give up his old identity and open himself to a new one. He has to will himself to have no will. Just as in the description of transformation of identity, there is a necessity for the individual to be active, to actively seek a state in which he no longer exists, a state of 'positive passivity': 'passiones[21]'. This necessity underlies the prayer in a pamphlet at Burrswood.

> Let us by an act of will, place ourselves in the presence of our Divine Lord, and, with an act of faith, ask that he will empty us of self, and of all desire sure that his most blessed will be done

and was expressed in a sermon at the ecumenical healing centre in these terms: 'You and I must empty ourselves and make ourselves open to the power and love of the risen healing Christ.'

The state of transcendence has therefore to be actively sought. As I argued for transformation of identity, and the two processes are interrelated, it is essential that the individual be involved in the leap to a new identity[22]. Nonetheless the process is not a simple one where the individual decides to give up his identity, particularly as he has to give up his bodily identity, which is pre-symbolic. To give up a bodily identity necessitates a weakening of the body image. The complete process thus has many of the characteristics of mind reform or brainwashing (see Frank, 1963; Lifton, 1963; Sargant, 1959; Schein, 1971). The body image of a sick person is already weak. This is of course especially true of those who are likely to consult healers, the chronic sick and the incurable. This weak body is then further assaulted. At Lourdes and other shrines this assault is the journey to the shrine itself, which exhausts the pilgrim[23]. Other techniques such as fasting may be used, e.g., the three-day fast imposed by the Health Centre. The effect of such assaults upon the body is the lowering of body blood sugar levels which reduces mental alertness and produces a tendency to blur reality and to hallucinate, in short to enter a trance state (see Abrahamson and Pezet, 1951; Gray Walter, 1953; Sargant, 1959).

Coupled with these direct assaults upon the body there are often 'attacks' upon the senses of the afflicted. Such 'attacks' can take two forms. The afflicted individual can be exposed to a sensory bombardment. This bombardment is achieved at Lourdes for example by the colour, music and ritual of the pilgrimage processions and masses. This produces sensory overload, an overload the more extreme because many sick people have withdrawn from the normal intensive stimuli of everyday life. This sensory overload may produce a state of transcendence. On the other hand the same effect can be achieved by sensory deprivation as the series of experiments at McGill University in the 1950s demonstrated (Bexton et al., 1954; Heron et al., 1956; Scott et al., 1959). These experiments demonstrated that people deprived of sensory input reported a sense of 'otherness' and a sense of 'bodily strangeness', they had distortions of their perception of space and they were more suggestible. The Health Centre (Chapter 5) utilises the technique of sensory deprivation when it deprives its new clients of any telephone, newspapers, radio, television or books (excepting the Bible and the book of the founder of the Centre). At the same time individuals are on a fast which lowers their body blood sugar levels.

This use of several different methods at once is normal in those processes of healing that seek transcendence. It seems likely that each method reinforces the other and that individuals who are prone to hallucination because of exhaustion, when their senses are bombarded or deprived in addition, are more likely to enter a trance state than those who are merely exhausted. It must be remembered also that people with low blood sugar levels are more open to suggestion and that people who are sensory deprived are open to suggestion. Both these factors may also reinforce each other, an important point when considering that healers not only seek to break down old identities but to build up new identities.

Taking people on journeys, making them fast and bombarding their senses with a high mass or depriving their senses of normal stimuli by banning the mass media are not the only techniques for producing transcendence. They are however the major ones I observed. In primitive societies other modes of reaching the same state are used extensively. Three in particular deserve special attention because of their ubiquity: dancing, music and drugs (see e.g. Kiev, 1966a). Dancing has the function of exhausting the participants and it is worth noting that most dancing in which the individual ultimately enters a trance state goes on all day and/or all night. Music seems to be important not only as another mode of providing a sensory bombardment but also as a direct means, through drumming, of inducing a trance state[24]. Finally drugs not only blur reality but appear to have the effect of short-circuiting the neurological mechanisms that control sensory input thus producing sensory overload (Zaehner, 1972).

One of the main methods of bombarding the senses of sick people is the use of ritual. This is not however just a question of volume. It is true that rituals, such as those at Lourdes, involve swirling movement, bright colours, repetitive music and chanting, all of which contribute to a sensory overload. In addition, however, they are multi-media message systems (Prince, 1964). One such message system has already been studied at Lourdes, but it is important to note that all rituals carry the 'message' that the normal orientations of time and space do not apply (Leach, 1976). This means that in so far as the afflicted individual is immersed in the ritual it breaks down the normal perceptual framework by which he locates himself in time and space. Now it appears that these basic perceptual concepts have a profound effect upon an individual if they are shattered or shifted. For example one researcher put a subject in deep hypnosis and then informed her that an oscillator she could hear was operating at a constant speed. In fact the speed was gradually stepped up with the result that the hypnotized subject became more and more manic. When the speed of the oscillator was gradually decreased the subject became depressed until she became catatonic as the oscillator came to rest. Such work suggests, as the person reporting it states, that a 'person's mood, emotion and cognition can be altered very radically through basic manipulation of the dimensions of time' (Sacerdote, 1977, p.312). As previous arguments have demonstrated a change in 'mood, emotion and cognition' can produce a change in bodily state, and Sacerdote for example claims to have cured people by eliciting in them experiences produced by hypnosis that were either of a kind that restricted perception or 'multi sensory experience involving expansion of space and time'. Such multi sensory experiences involving expansion of space and time are precisely what successful rituals achieve.

As with the process of transformation so with the processes that elicit transcendence: it is not a simple matter of applying them to the afflicted individual. There is an interaction between the individual and the experience. This interaction and the problems involved in trying to analyse it, can be demonstrated by looking at the fact that the majority of those cured at Lourdes are women and peasants. Why should this be the case? There are several arguments that might explain it. Firstly there is the simple fact that the majority of pilgrims to Lourdes over the last century have been women and peasants. These are the most religious categories of society and are more likely to go on a pilgrimage. Their preponderance may thus be a 'demographic fact' as the head of the Bureau Medicale expressed it to me in interview. Second, peasants, and women (and women peasants in particular) normally live isolated lives with a limited sensory input. Lourdes may therefore more readily be a sensory overload to those whose social isolation may be broken only by a weekly trip to a local market where most faces are familiar. In Lourdes they are faced with a vast number of strangers and new experiences all of which must create difficulties in assimilation. Third, their identity may be of a different nature than that of town dwellers.

There are two arguments involved here. It may be that peasants have a lesser individuality than town dwellers as Blum and Blum (1965, p.42) suggest of Greek peasants:

> Reared as he had been and will be, in such a manner that being with and part of others is his only experience he has little 'private self' that allows him to objectify what is physically and emotionally his view; what is another's...The personality, the self of the child, is formed not just by associating with others but by merging with them...For him being alone is loneliness, and loneliness is terror, for without the company of others he feels part of himself is gone.

Such an 'other directed' individual (Riesman et al., 1950)

is more likely to change under the social pressures and
expectations of a pilgrimage event than an 'inner directed'
town dweller. It may be also that peasants do not only have
an identity that merges with others but one that merges with
the cosmos as well. Peasant consciousness, Manning and
Fabrega (1973) suggest, is one where their self, their body,
their interpersonal relations and nature are all seen as
existing in a continuity. Like the characters in
Shakespeare's plays or the people living in the world
described by Keith Thomas (1973) they expect a change in the
cosmos to be reflected in their social world and in their
bodies. Such individuals when they experience a fundamental
shift in their experience of the cosmos, in their perception
of space and time, may well experience a concomitant shift
in their bodies to maintain this continuity. In this respect
the fourth and final argument may be important - peasants
know and understand the ritual forms of the pilgrimage.
Their initial identity is closely bound up with the initial
view of the cosmos, a view transcended in the experience of
transcendence in which they have no identity and from which
they move to a new identity bound up with a new view of the
cosmos expressed in the messages of the ritual.

All this is however speculative. The precise interaction
between the identity the individual brings to the healer or
healing process, the experience of transcendence and the new
identity that those successfully healed emerge with is an
area that needs much further research. What I want to
suggest strongly here is that such an investigation should
focus on the experience of transcendence. It is itself a
factor in making an individual adopt a new identity. It is a
highly unusual experience and one that cannot be easily
communicated. In such a situation individuals become very
dependent on those who appear to understand it and those who
provide an explanation are often given exaggerated powers
(Light, 1978b). The granting of such powers is of course
extremely important in effecting a change in identity as the
literature on placebo reaction and the arguments earlier in
the chapter on transformation stress. What appears to be
happening when instantaneous cures are recorded is that the
afflicted individual, subjected to the full gamut of
techniques, as at Lourdes, is disorientated through
physiological means, through sensory overload and through
the breakdown of his perceptual framework. The framework of
his body, the framework of his senses and the cultural
framework with respect to such basic concepts as time and
space are all subject to attack. His old identity, his old
way of looking at the world, is completely destroyed and he
experiences transcendence in which he loses all his old
identities, both social and animal. In this state he is
extremely suggestible, a blank sheet on which a new identity
can be built. That building has already taken place. The new
identity is waiting for him. The pilgrim from the time he
decides to go on a pilgrimage has been presented with a new
identity and the process of pilgrimage may be seen as an
assertion of that identity. Similarly the healer from the
first time he meets a client is engaged in providing a new

identity for the client. The processes of transformation have already provided a new identity. The individual only becomes aware of that new identity at the 'turning point' and he then re-interprets his former experience and sees it as leading to his present change in identity[25].

Transformation and transcendence are interlinked. It is possible to have transformation of identity without transcendence, which is the normal process of healing. It produces symptom relief. However it is not possible to have transcendence as part of a healing process without transformation. The processes of transformation, which may include ritual, provide the individual with a new identity which when he experiences the state of no-identity, transcendence, provides him with a ready-made identity to step into, an identity as a healthy functioning individual.

NOTES

(1) Young (1976) discusses this and Turner (1968) and Harwood (1970) give excellent examples of it.

(2) Kleinman and Sung (1976). Also see the work of Pattison and his colleagues (1973) who from their study of a pentecostal sect came to the conclusion that 'the subject's perception of healing was related to their participation in a healing ritual, not a perception of change in symptomatology (and) from the subject's point of view, relief of symptoms is really a tangential issue. For them faith healing reaffirms their belief system and their style of life.'

(3) It is worth noting that many of those who draw the distinction between organic, psychological and social aspects of affliction are themselves medical practitioners as well as anthropologists.

(4) My discussion of these philosophical questions is obviously hesitant and incomplete. My understandings come from a symposium on the mind/body problem held at the University of McGill in February 1978 at which neurobiologists, psychologists and philosophers gave papers and from several books and articles: Austin (1970); Bateson (1972); Bertalanffy (1964); Black (1969); Graham (1967); Gray Walter (1953); Mandler (1975); Perry (1975); Phillips (1934); Ryle (1949); Van Peursen (1966); Wilkes (1978); Wittkower (1969).

(5) Why they are so constructed is an interesting question. Stent (1978) argues that it is because of evolutionary development.

(6) This model is derived from various sources but the major inspiration is the work of Ernst Becker (1971).

(7) A view I share with Freud.

(8) See Schachter and Singer (1962) for an experiment which demonstrates this.

(9) See Kiev (1964); Lewis (1975); Turner (1963 and 1968) for tribal societies and Blum and Blum (1965); Holland and Tharp (1964); Manning and Fabrega (1973) and Nash (1967) for peasant societies.

(10) I have oversimplified the actual process here for ease

of exposition: There is extensive evidence (see e.g. Blum and Blum, 1965; Maclean, 1971; Schwartz, 1969) that there is a 'hierarchy of resort' in which unorthodox healers are called in for some illnesses and not for others and at some stages of illness but not at others.

(11) The authoritative nature of the healer's role has been noted by Fabrega (1970), Kiev (1966b), Larner (1976), and Prince (1964). Also Modarressi (1966) noted that healers in South Iran are called 'Father' to symbolise an authoritative, close and enduring relationship.

(12) A good account of the use of science in impression management is provided in Cowie and Roebuck's (1975) account of a chiropractic clinic.

(13) Romano (1965) suggests that upper-class patronage is important in promoting the fame of a healer. It is being suggested here that it is also an important aspect of his authority, an authority essential for the healing process.

(14) Lubchansky et al. (1970) stress the same point in their study of Puerto Rican spiritualists: '...spiritualists tend to use short sentences and to take pains to use the exact terminology of the patient, accepting his symptoms exactly as they are described.'

(15) Hospital chaplain involved in healing, in interview.

(16) Harry Edwards, see Chapter 2.

(17) A man who had helped set up the ecumenical healing centre.

(18) Other methods that can be used for this purpose such as the self-help groups (Bumbalo and Young, 1973) typical of Alcholics Anonymous or the class-groups of Charles Wesley were not evident in the healers I studied.

(19) Sermon at Lourdes.

(20) Letter in Letter 74, Christmas 1973, London Healing Mission.

(21) See Lienhardt (1961) for the development of the idea of passiones.

(22) Donald Light (1978a) makes a similar point in regard to the training of psychiatrists when he says 'if a program wishes to break down old values and ways of seeing the world, it will maximise involvement or responsibility as well as heighten a feeling of uncertainty'.

(23) One of the reasons for the reduced number of miracles in recent years may be the advent of the aeroplane.

(24) See Neher's, 1962, experiment with drum beats.

(25) The parallels with detailed analyses of conversion are numerous. e.g. see Hine (1969), Goodman et al. (1974) and Van Zandt (1977).

Bibliography

Abrahamson, E.M. and Pezet, A.W. (1951) Body, Mind and Sugar, Holt, Rinehart and Winston, New York.
Academy of Parapsychology and Medicine (1972) The Dimensions of Healing: A Symposium, Los Altos, California.
Austin, J.L. (1970) 'Intelligent Behaviour' in Ryle eds, O.P. Wood and G. Pitcher, Macmillan.
Bateson, G. (1972) Steps to an Ecology of Mind, Ballantine Books, New York.
Becker, E. (1971) The Birth and Death of Meaning, Penguin.
Beecher, H.K. (1955) 'The Powerful Placebo', Journal of the American Medical Association, 24.
Bernard, H. (1975) Une Reponse a L'Alienation des Malades et Infirmes, Oratoire St. Joseph du Mont-Royal, Montreal.
Bertalanffy, L. von (1964) 'The Mind Body Problem: a New View', Psychosomatic Medicine, Jan-Feb.
Bexton, W.H., Heron, W., and Scott T.H. (1954) 'Effects of Decreased Variation in the Sensory Environment', Canadian Journal of Psychology, 8, 2.
Bindra, (1976) A Theory of Intelligent Behaviour, Wiley.
Black, S. (1969) Mind and Body, Wm. Kimber.
Blanton, S. (1940) 'Analytic Study of a Cure at Lourdes', Psychoanalytic Quarterly, 384-'62.
Blum, R. and Blum A. (1965) Health and Healing in Rural Greece, Stanford University Press, California.
Buber, M. (1947) Between Man and Man, Routledge and Kegan Paul Ltd.
Bumbalo, J.A. and Young, D.E. (1973) 'The Self Help Phenomenon'. American Journal of Nursing, 73, 9.
Cade, M. and Coxhead, N. (1979) The Awakened Mind, Wildwood House.
Calestro, K. (1972) 'Psychotherapy, Faith Healing and Suggestion', International Journal of Psychiatry, 10. 2.
Cartwright, A. and O'Brien, M. (1978) 'Social class variations in health care and in the nature of general practice consultations', in Basic Readings in Medical Sociology, eds. D. Tuckett and G.M. Kaufert, Tavistock.
Chertok, I. (1969) 'Psychosomatic Medicine in the West and in Eastern European Countries', Psychosomatic Medicine, 31.
Clark, M. (1970) Health in the Mexican-American Culture, University of California Press.

Clogg, C.C. (1978) 'The Effects of Personal Health Care upon Longevity in an Economically Advanced Population', unpublished paper read at the 1978 conference of the American Sociological Association, San Francisco.

Cobb, S. (1976) 'Social Support as a Moderator of Life Stress'. Psychosomatic Medicine, 38, 5.

Colson, A.B. (1976) 'Binary Oppositions and the Treatment of Sickness among the Akawaio', in Social Anthropology and Medicine, ed. J.B. Loudon. Association of Social Anthropologists of the Commonwealth, Monograph 13.

Comaroff, J. (1976) 'A Bitter Pill to Swallow: Placebo theory in General Practice', Sociological Review, 24.

Coulthard, M. and Ashby, M. (1976) 'A Linguistic Description of Doctor-Patient Interviews'. In Studies in Everyday Medical Life, eds. M. Wadsworth and D. Robinson, published by Martin Robertson.

Cowie, J.B. and Roebuck, J. (1975) An Ethnography of a Chiropractic Clinic, Free Press.

Cruickshank, W.M. (1948) 'The Impact of Physical Disability on Social Adjustment', Journal of Social Issues, 4, 4.

Delgado, R. (1969) Physical Control of the Mind, Harper Colophon, New York.

Demetrio, F.R. (1970) Dictionary of Philippine Folk Beliefs and Customs, Xavier University, Cagayan de Oro City, Library of Congress, Number 78-150504.

Douglas, M. (1970) Purity and Danger, Pelican.

Douglas, M. (1973) Natural Symbols, Barrie and Jackson.

Dunlop, D.W. (1975) 'Alternatives to "Modern" Health Delivery Systems in Africa: Public Policy Issues of Traditional Health Systems', Social Science and Medicine, 9, 11/12, 581-586.

Eagle, R. (1978) Alternative Medicine, Futura.

Edwards, H. (1968) Harry Edwards: Thirty Years a Spiritual Healer, The Healer Publishing Company Ltd., Burrows Lea, Shere, Surrey.

Eisenberg, L. (1977) 'Disease and Illness: Distinction between Professional and Popular Ideas of Sickness', Culture, Medicine and Psychiatry, 1, 1.

Eliade, M. (1964) Shamanism, Princeton University Press.

Evans-Pritchard, E.E. (1937) Witchcraft, Oracles and Magic among the Azande, Oxford University Press.

Fabrega, H. (1970) 'Dynamics of Medical Practice in a Folk Community', Millbank Memorial Fund Quarterly,, 48, 391-412.

Fabrega, H. and Silver, D.B. (1973) Illness and Shamanistic Curing in Zinacantan, Stanford University Press.

Field, D. (1976) 'The Social Definition of Illness', in An Introduction to Medical Sociology, ed. D. Tucket, published by Tavistock.

Finucane, R.C. (1977) Miracles and Pilgrims, Dent.

Fisher, H.K. and Olin, B.M. (1956) 'The Dynamics of Placebo Therapy: A Clinical Study', American Journal of Medical Science, 232, 504-512.

Fisher, S. and Cleveland, S.E. (1968) Body Image and Personality, Dover Publications Inc., New York.

Foster, G.M. (1965) 'Peasant Society and the Image of the Limited Good', American Anthropologist, 67.

Frank, J.D. (1963) _Persuasion ahd Healing_, Schocken Books, New York.

Frankenberg, R. and Leeson, J. (1976) 'Disease, Illness and Sickness: Social Aspects of the Choice of Healer in a Lusaka Suburb', in _Social Anthropology and Medicine_, ed. J. Loudon, A.S.A.C. Monograph 13.

Gelfand, M. (1964) 'Psychiatric Disorders as Recognised by the Shona', in _Magic, Faith and Healing_, Free Press, New York, ed. A. Kiev.

Goffman, E. (1956) 'The Nature of Deference and Demeanor', _American Anthropologist_, 58.

Goffman, E. (1968) _Stigma_, Penguin.

Goffman, E. (1971) _Asylums_, Penguin.

Goodman, F.D. et al. (1974) _Trance, Healing and Hallucination_, Wiley.

Grad, B. et al. (1961) 'An Unorthodox Method of Treament on Wound Healing in Mice', _International Journal of Parapsychology_, 3, 5-24.

Grad, B. (1967) 'The Laying on of Hands: Implications for Psychotherapy, Gentling and the Placebo Effect', _Journal of the American Society for Psychical Research_, 61, 4.

Graham, D.T. (1967) 'Health, Disease and the Mind-Body Problem: Linguistic Parallelism', _Psychosomatic Medicine_, 29, 52-71.

Gray Walter, W. (1953) _The Living Brain_, Norton, New York.

Happold, F.C. (1963) _Mysticism_, Pelican.

Harwood, A. (1970) _Witchcraft, Sorcery and Social Categories among the Safwa_, Oxford University Press.

Heron, W., Doane, B.K. and Scott, T.H. 'Visual Disturbance after Prolonged Perceptual Isolation', _Canadian Journal of Psychology_, 10, 13-18.

Hessler, R.M. (1975) 'Intra Ethnic Diversity: Health Care of the Chinese Americans, _Human Organisation_, 34, Fall.

Hine, V.H. (1969) 'Pentecostal Glossolalia', _Journal for the Scientific Study of Religion_, 8.

Holland, W.R. and Tharp, R.G. (1964) 'Highland Maya Psychotherapy', _American Anthropologist_, 66, 41-52.

Illich, I. (1974) _Medical Nemesis: The Expropriation of Health_, Calder and Boyars.

Ingham, J. (1975) 'On Mexican Folk Medicine', _American Anthropologist_, 72.

Jospe, M. (1978) _The Placebo Effect in Healing_, Lexington Books, Massachusetts.

Katz, M.S. (1972) _Chiropractic - A Faith Healing Business._ Presented to the Hearings on the Chiropractic Act, Canada.

Kessel, L. (1959) 'Spontaneous Disappearance of Bilateral Pulmonary Metastases', _Journal of the American Medical Association_, 169, 15.

Kiev, A. (1966a) 'The Psychotherapeutic Value of Spirit Possession on Haiti', in _Trance and Possession States_, ed. R. Prince, published by the R.M. Bucke Memorial Society, Montreal.

Kiev, A. (1966b) 'Obstacles to Medical Progress in Haiti', _Human Organisation_, 25, 10-15.

Kimball, C.P. (1970) 'Conceptual Developments in Psychosomatic Medicine 1939-1969', _Annals of Internal Medicine_, 73.

Kingston, J. (1975) Healing Without Medicine, Aldus Books.
Kleinman, A.M. (1973) 'Some Issues for a Comparative Study of Medical Healing', International Journal of Social Psychiatry, 19, 159-165.
Kleinman, A. and Sung, L.H. (1976) 'Why do Indigenous Practitioners Successfully Heal?', Social Science and Medicine, vol. 13B, 1, 1979.
Klopfer, B. (1957) 'Psychological Variables in Human Cancer', Journal of Projective Techniques, 21.
Krieger, D. (19756) 'Therapeutic Touch: The Imprimatur of Nursing', American Journal of Nursing, 75, 5.
Kuhn, T.S. (1962) The Structure of Scientific Revolutions, University of Chicago Press.
Ladieu, G., Alder, D.L. and Dembo, T. (1948) 'Studies in Adjustment to Visible Injuries: Social Acceptance of the Injured', Journal of Social Issues, 4, 4.
Laing, R.D. (1971) Self and Others, Pelican.
Lambourne, R.A. (1963) Community, Church and Healing, Darton, Longman and Todd.
LaPatra, J. (1978) Healing, McGraw Hill, New York.
Larner, K. (1976) 'Healing in Pre-Industrial Britain', unpublished paper given at the British Sociological Association Conference.
Lasagna, L. et al. (1954) 'A Study of the Placebo Response', American Journal of Medicine, 16, 770-779.
Leach, E. (1976 Culture and Communication, Cambridge University Press.
Lederer, H.D. (1965) 'How the Sick View their World', in Social Interaction and Patient Care, eds. J.K. Skipper and R.G. Leonard, published by J.B. Lipincott, Philadelphia.
Lee, R.B. (1968) 'The Sociology of Kung Bushman Trance Performances' in Trance and Possession States, ed. R. Prince, published by R.M. Bucke Memorial Society, Montreal.
Lewis, A.J. (1953) 'Health as a Social Concept', British Journal of Sociology, 4, 109-124.
Lewis, G. (1975) Knowledge of Illness in a Sepik Society, Athlone Press, University of London, L.S.E. Monograph 52.
Lieban, R.W. (1965) 'Shamanism and Social Control in a Philippine City', Journal of the Folklore Institute, 2, 443-454.
Lieban, R.W. (1966) 'Fatalism and Medicine in Cebuana Areas of the Philippines', Anthropological Quarterly, 39, 171-179.
Lieban, R.W. (1967) Cebuana Sorcery, University of California Press.
Lienhardt, G. (1961) Divinity and Experience, Oxford University Press.
Lifton, R.J. (1963) Thought Reform and the Psychology of Totalism, Norton, New York.
Light, D. (1978a) 'The Moral Career of the Psychiatric Resident', unpublished paper available Department of Community Medicine, Mt. Sinai School of Medicine, New York.
Light, D. (1978b) 'Uncertainty and Control in Professional Training', unpublished paper given at the A.S.A. Conference, San Francisco. Published in 1979 in Journal of Health and Social Behaviour, vol. 20, 310-322.

Lipowski, Z.J. (1969) 'Psychosocial Aspects of Disease', Annals of Internal Medicine, 71, 6.

Lubchansky, I., Egri, G. and Stokes, I. (1970) 'Puerto Rican Spiritualists View Mental Illness, American Journal of Psychiatry, 127, 312-321.

Ludwig, A.M. (1968) 'Altered States of Consciousness', in Trance and Possession States, ed. R. Prince, published by the R.M. Bucke Memorial Society, Montreal.

Lyons, J. (1970) Chomsky, Fontana Modern Masters.

Malinowski, B. (1954) Magic, Science and Religion, Doubleday, New York.

Mandler, G. (1975) Mind and Emotion, Wiley.

Manning, P.K. and Fabrega, H. (1973) 'The Experience of Self and Body: Health and Illness in the Chiapas Highlands', in Phenomenological Sociology, ed. G. Psathas, published by Wiley.

Mathers, J. (1970) 'Psychiatry and Religion', in Religion and Medicine: A Discussion, ed. M.A.H. Melinsky, SCM Press.

Mead, G.H. (1977) 'The Self', in Modern Sociology: Introductory Readings, ed. P. Worsley, published by Penguin.

Millman, M. (1977) The Unkindest Cut, Wm. Morrow and Co., New York.

Mischel, F. (1959) 'Faith Healing and Medical Practice in the Southern Caribbean', Southwest Journal of Anthropology, 15, 407-417.

Modarressi, T. (1966) 'The Zar Cult in South Iran', in Trance and Possession States, ed. R. Prince, published by the R.M. Bucke Memorial Society, Montreal.

MacLean, U. (1971) Magical Medicine, Allen Lane.

McNutt, F. (1974) Healing, Fowler Wright Books, Tunbridge Wells.

Nash, J. (1967) 'The Logic of Behaviour: Curing in a Maya Indian Town', Human Organisation, 26.

Neher, A. (1962) 'A Physiological Explanation of Unusual Behaviour in Ceremonies Involving Drums', Human Biology, 4, 151-160.

New, P.K. (1977) 'Traditional and Modern Health Care: An Appraisal of Complementarity, International Social Science Journal, 29, 3.

New, P.K. and New, M.L. (1975) 'The Links Between Health and the Political Structure in New China', Human Organisation, 34, 3.

New, P.K. and New, M.L. (1977) 'The Barefoot Doctors of China', in Culture, Disease and Healing, ed. D. Landy, published by Collier Macmillan.

Parker, G. and Tupling, H. (1976) 'The Chiropractic Patient: Psychosocial Aspects', The Medical Journal of Australia, 2, 10.

Parsinnen, T.M. (1979) 'Professional Deviants and the History of Medicine: Medical Mesmerists in Victorian Britain', in Wallis, R. (ed.), On the Margins of Science, Soc. Review Monograph 27, University of Keele.

Pattison, E., Lapins, N. and Doerr, H. 'Faith Healing: A Study of Personality and Function, Journal of Nervous and Mental Disease, 157, 6.

Perry, J. (1975) Personal Identity, University of California Press.

Phillips, R.P. (1934) Modern Thomist Philosophy, Volume 1. Burns, Oates and Washbourne.

Press, I. (1969) 'Urban Illness: Physicians, Curers and Dual Use in Bogota', Journal of Health and Social Behaviour, 10, 3.

Press, I. (1971) 'The Urban Curandero', American Anthropologist, 73, 741-756.

Press, I. (1978) 'Urban Folk Medicine: A Functional Overview', American Anthropologist, 80, 1.

Prince, R. (1964) 'Indigenous Yoruba Psychiatry', in Magic, Faith and Healing, ed. A. Kiev, published by Free Press, New York.

Prince, R. (1972) 'Fundamental Differences of Psychoanalysis and Faith Healing', International Journal of Psychiatry, 10, 2.

Rebsomen, A. (1930) Cinquante Ans D'Hospitalite, 1880-1930, Editions Spes., Paris.

Renneker, R. and Cutler, M. (1952) 'Psychological Problems of Adjustment to Cancer of the Breast', Journal of the American Medical Association, 148.

Reyner, J.H., Laurence, G. and Upton, C. (1974) Psionic Medicine, Routledge and Kegan Paul Ltd.

Riesman, D. et al. (1950) The Lonely Crowd, Yale University Press, New Haven.

Riley, T.N. and Semsri, S. (1974) 'The Variegated Thai Medical System as a Context for Birth Control Services', Working Paper No. 6, Institute for Population and Social Research, Mahadol University, 420/1 Rajuithi, Phayathai, Bangkok, 4, Thailand.

Romano, O.I. (1965) 'Charismatic Medicine, Folk Healing and Folk Sainthood', American Anthropologist, 67, 1151-1173.

Rosenfeld, A. (1975) The Second Genesis, Vintage Books, New York.

Roth, J.A. (1963) Timetables, Bobbs-Merrill.

Ryle, G. (1949) The Concept of Mind, Hutchinson.

Sacerdote, P. (1977) 'Applications of Hypnotically Elicited Mystical States to the Treatment of Physical and Emotional Pain', International Journal of Clinical and Experimental Hypnosis, 25, 4.

Sargant, W. (1959) Battle for the Mind, Pan.

Schachter, S. and Singer, J.E. (1962) 'Cognitive, Social and Physiological Determinants of Emotional State', Psychological Review, 69, 5.

Schein, E.H. (1971) Coercive Persuasion, Norton Library, U.S.A.

Schwartz, L.R. (1969) 'The Hierarchy of Resort in Curative Practices: The Admiralty Islands, Melanesia, Journal of Health and Social Behaviour, 10, 201-220.

Scott, T.H., Bexton, W.H., Heron, W. and Doane, B.K. (1959) 'Cognitive Effects of Perceptual Isolation', Canadian Journal of Psychology, 13, 3.

Shapiro, A.K. (1964) 'Factors Contributing to the Placebo Effect', American Journal of Psychotherapy, 18 (supplement 1), 73-88.

Skultans, V. (1974) Intimacy and Ritual, Routledge and Kegan Paul Ltd.

Smith, J.M. (1972) 'Paranormal Effects on Enzyme Activity', Human Decisions, 1, 15-19.

Spraggett, A. (1970) Kathryn Kuhlman, The Woman Who Believes in Miracles, T.Y. Crowell, Inc.

Stent, G.S. (1978) Paradoxes of Progress, W.H. Freeman and Co., San Francisco.

Strauss, A. (1959) Mirrors and Masks: The Search for Identity, Free Press.

Sutherland, A.M. and Orbach, C.E. (1953) 'Depressive Reactions Associated with Surgery for Cancer', in Psychological Aspects of Cancer, The American Cancer Society.

Szasz, T.S. and Hollander, M.H. (1956) 'A Contribution to the Philosophy of Medicine', A.M.A. Archives of Internal Medicine, 95, 585-592.

Tajon, R.V. (undated) Alex Orbito, Exponent of Spiritual Therapy, World Mission Society, P.O. Box 4388, Manilla, Philippines.

Thomas, K. (1973) Religion and the Decline of Magic, Penguin.

Topley, M. (1970) 'Chinese Traditional Ideas and the Treatment of Disease: Two Examples from Hong Kong', Man, 5, 421-437.

Tuckett, D. (1976) An Introduction to Medical Sociology, Tavistock.

Turner, R.H. (1976) 'The Real Self: From Institution to Impulse', American Journal of Sociology, 81, 5.

Turner, V.W. (1963) The Forest of Symbols, Cornell University Press.

Turner, V.W. (1968) The Drums of Affliction, Clarendon Press, Oxford.

Turner, V.W. (1974a) The Ritual Process, Pelican.

Turner, V.W. (1974b) 'Pilgrimages as Social Processes', in Drama, Fields and Metaphors, ed. V.W. Turner, published by Cornell University Press.

Turner, V.W. (1974c) 'Social Dramas and Ritual Metaphors', ibid.

Turner, V.W. and Turner, E. (1978) Image and Pilgrimage in Christian Culture, Columbia University Press, New York.

Van Peursen, C.A. (1966) Body, Soul and Spirit: A Survey of the Body-Mind Problem, Oxford University Press.

Van Zandt, D. (1977) 'Conversion and Interaction', unpublished paper given at the B.S.A. Sociology of Religion Study Group.

Webster, A.J. (1979) 'Scientific Controversy and Socio-Cognitive Metonymy: The Case of Acupuncture', in Wallis, R. (ed.), On the Margins of Science, University of Keele, Monograph 27.

White, R.K., Wright, A. and Dembo, T. (1948) 'Studies of Adjustment to Visible Injuries: Evaluation of Curiosity by the Injured, Journal of Abnormal and Social.Psychology, 43, 13-28.

Wilkes, K.V. (1978) Physicalism, Routledge and Kegan Paul Ltd.

Wilson, M. (1966) The Church is Healing, SCM Press.

Wittkower, E.D. et al. (1969) 'A Global Survey of Psychosomatic Medicine', International Journal of Psychiatry, 7, 1.

Wolf, S. (1950) 'Effects of Suggestion and Conditioning on the Action of Chemical Agents in Human Subjects - The Pharmacology of Placebos', Journal of Clinical Investigation, 29.

Wolf, S. and Pinsky, R.H. (1954) 'Effects of Placebo Administration and Occurrence of Toxic Reactions', Journal of the American Medical Association, 155, 339-341.

Wright, B.A. (1960) Physical Disability: A Psychological Approach, Harper and Row, New York.

Wright, P.W.G. (1979) 'A Study in the Legitimation of Knowledge. The "Success" of Medicine and the "Failure" of Astrology', in On the Margins of Science, ed. R. Wallis, Keele University, Monograph 27.

Young, A. (1976) 'Some Implications of Medical Beliefs and Practice for Social Anthropology', American Anthropologist, 78, 1.

Zaehner, R.C. (1972) Drugs, Mysticism and Make-Believe, Collins.

Index